NEW PERSPECTIVES IN HEALTH PROMOTION

This important book introduces the Health in All Policies (HiAP) approach to health promotion not only detailing how policymaking at all levels can foster the right conditions for better public health but also examining the inherent challenges to such an overarching approach.

Building on the author's extensive experience in health promotion planning in both regional and international contexts, the book recognizes those factors which influence public health outside of healthcare services themselves. Addressing these broader social, economic and even cultural issues, it discusses how policymaking between the public and private sectors, as well as local and national government, should be both collaborative and holistic. But the book also reflects upon the key difficulties in integrating multi-sector and multi-level approaches – both top-down and bottom-up policymaking – to create processes that further health equity and empower individuals and communities.

Now at the forefront of current thinking in health promotion and health policy, this insightful overview of HiAP will be essential reading for students and researchers across the Health Sciences, specifically Public Health and Social Policy, as well as every practitioner in the field.

Roar Amdam is Professor Emeritus in Planning and Leadership at Volda University College, Norway.

NEW PERSPECTIVES IN HEALTH PROMOTION

Health in All Policies (HiAP)

Roar Amdam

Routledge
Taylor & Francis Group
LONDON AND NEW YORK

Designed cover image: Getty

First published 2025
by Routledge
4 Park Square, Milton Park, Abingdon, Oxon OX14 4RN

and by Routledge
605 Third Avenue, New York, NY 10158

Routledge is an imprint of the Taylor & Francis Group, an informa business

British Library Cataloguing-in-Publication Data
A catalogue record for this book is available from the British Library

ISBN: 978-1-032-58735-6 (hbk)
ISBN: 978-1-032-58736-3 (pbk)
ISBN: 978-1-003-45127-3 (ebk)

DOI: 10.4324/9781003451273

Typeset in Times New Roman
by KnowledgeWorks Global Ltd.

CONTENTS

FIGURES AND TABLES

Figures

Tables

ABOUT THE AUTHOR

Professor emeritus **Roar Amdam** is full professor in planning and leadership at the Volda University College in Norway. He was head of the master's programme in planning and leadership at the college from 1999 to 2019. His major research question has been how to use planning as a tool in development of regions and local communities, organizations and public health work. Central themes in his research are innovation, collaboration, empowerment, capacity building and legitimacy. He has published several books and articles. He was awarded the Research Prize for 2021 at the University College of Volda.

PREFACE

When the book *Planning in Health Promotion Work – An Empowerment Model* was published in 2010, the content was mainly how I as a planning expert had advised an EU project aimed at integrating health considerations in spatial planning and development and contributing to sustainable public health in the Baltic Sea Region. In this situation, it became natural for me to summarize the knowledge and experiences we had from local and regional planning and development and to reflect on how to use this in public health. In accordance with the main goal of the HEPRO project, my role in the project became to develop and implement training programmes in public health work aimed at various target groups, to build understanding of spatial health planning and the use of local health profiles. The book discussed how the HEPRO project approach could be interpreted regarding the governance and communicative turn in planning, and also discussed the theoretical fundamentals of the planning model used in the HEPRO project and outlined the empowerment planning model which I later called the ISTOL model. Further the book discussed empowerment evaluation and showed how monitoring and evaluation could contribute to learning at different levels in the empowerment planning model. The book ended with some reflections.

Since then the Health in All Policies (HiAP) approach to public health has become dominant. This approach regards policymaking as a multi-actor process with planning and partnerships as tools, but HiAP seems to lack institutional capacity and democratic legitimacy. However, handling the COVID-19 pandemic in Norway and in other countries became HiAP in practice with enough legitimacy and capacity to succeed. Therefore, I argue in this updated book in favour of handling public health issues in a similar way the COVID-19 pandemic was handled. This updated book has six chapters, and all chapters have content from the first book, but the content is reorganized, shortened, supplemented and rewritten to build a chain of argument leading up to a conclusion that HiAP need to be practised as radical New Public Governance.

1

PERSPECTIVES IN HEALTH IN ALL POLICIES

In this chapter, Health in All Policies (HiAP) is interpreted as a multi-actor collaborative process with a pragmatic approach to theory and practice, and this chapter presents an overview of central terms used to understand and explain the complexity of HiAP and the challenges this form of public health work is facing regarding planning, participation, partnerships and policymaking. The next chapters discuss the challenges more in detail; how to handle them and the prerequisites for successful HiAP practice.

Introduction

About hundred years ago, public health was defined as a top-down activity:

> … the science and the art of preventing disease, prolonging life, and promoting physical health and efficiency through organized community efforts for the sanitation of the environment, the control of community infections, the education of the individual in principles of personal hygiene, the organization of medical and nursing service for the early diagnosis and preventive treatment of disease, and the development of the social machinery which will ensure to every individual in the community a standard of living adequate for the maintenance of health.
>
> (Winslow, 1920: 30)

Much later, the World Health Organization (1986) in the Ottawa Charter defined the purpose of public health as a bottom-up process of enabling people to increase control over their health and its determinants. The background for this new definition was the traditional shortcomings of public health services which

DOI: 10.4324/9781003451273-1

often undermined the clients' sense of capacity and self-worth and reduced their involvement in their own health (Huang & Wang, 2005: 13). These definitions imply that public health is a combination of top-down and bottom-up politics:

- to improve the health of populations by keeping people healthy, improve their health and prevent disease, and
- to improve individual and collective capacity to take healthy actions and the perceptions of the quality of living in the context they live.

Empowerment strategies, participation, community development and other bottom-up approaches have become important in public health, this in contrast to the top-down strategies that still dominated the 1960s and 1970s (Wold & Mittelmark, 2018; Kokko, Liveng & Torp, 2018). According to Kickbusch (2003) since the 1980s public administration leaders, health professionals, non-government agencies, government agencies, etc. have increasingly turned to empowerment and community participation as major strategies for alleviating poverty and social exclusion and reducing health disparities. Thus, public health has become a complex, dynamic and comprehensive policymaking process. It is a multi-level and multi-sector approach involving individuals, communities, stats, etc. and public, private and voluntary sector in governing structures and processes. Public health, as a community development process, has become a territory-based and multi-actor approach that uses *planning, participation, partnership* and *policymaking* to support and increase the inhabitants' and communities' ability to solve their own problems. In this new approach, individuals need competence to take more responsibility for their own health and well-being and communities need capacity and legitimacy to implement sustainable HiAP (Amdam, 2023).

The Health in All Policies approach

The HiAP practice of public health assumes that both individuals and communities must take more responsibility for their own health and well-being and that public health work must become an area for cooperation between several sectors and levels of government (Castro et al., 2016). HiAP is commonly regarded as an approach to public health policies that systematically draw upon a recognition that factors outside of healthcare services determine our health and that health decisions must be made across sectors at all levels of policymaking to improve population health and health equity. HiAP represents a collaborative approach that articulates health considerations and integrates them into policymaking, both vertically within different government authorities and horizontally between the public, private and voluntary sectors, with the mission to improve the health of all communities and all people. The HiAP approach is adopted in national politics worldwide, but it appears to be little literature on how to implement HiAP locally (Guglielmin et al., 2018), which is the subject of this book.

Public health issues are often regarded as ungovernable and wicked problems that need sharing knowledge and collaboration in networks (Weber & Khademian, 2008). The common characteristic for these problems is that they are complex, stubborn and unruly and that it is the inhabitants who create them, and that they consequently are part of the solution (Rittel & Webber, 1973; Rose, 1979; Schiefloe, 2021). Therefore, HiAP as a multi-actor and inter-sector collaboration depends on the inhabitants and the different actors from government sectors and levels' willingness and ability to collaborate. Therefore, the HiAP approach is not self-evident, and the approach is not easily implemented neither at global nor at local level.

The World Health Organization has played a significant role in promoting the public health approaches (Ståhl, 2018; Weber, 2020). In the Declaration of Alma Ata, the full participation of the community in the multi-dimensional work of health improvement became one of the pillars of the public health promotion and the Health to all movement (World Health Organization, 1978). The first International Conference on Health Promotion was held in Ottawa in 1986 and in the Ottawa Charter, the purposes of health promotion are formulated as a process of enabling people to increase their control over and to improve their health (World Health Organization, 1986). Since then, the World Health Organization Global Health Promotion Conferences have established and developed the global principles and action areas for health promotion. Community empowerment, planning and participation are in the Sundsvall Statement on Supportive Environments for Health seen as important factors in health promotion approach and the driving force for self-reliance and development (World Health Organization, 1991). And according to the Jakarta Declaration (World Health Organization, 1997), breaking down barriers between sectors and levels and creating partnerships were seen as essential for health promotion. These partnerships for health promotion were defined as voluntary agreements between two or more partners to work cooperatively towards a set of shared health outcomes. This broad approach to health was enforced in the Helsinki statement HiAP (World Health Organization, 2013) when health promotion was described as a collaborative approach that articulates health considerations and integrates them into policymaking. Most recently, the Ninth Global Conference in Shanghai 2016 highlighted the critical links between promoting health and the 2030 Agenda for Sustainable Development (World Health Organization, 2017) and made public health mainstream through the United Nations' 2030 Sustainable Development Goals (SDG) initiative.

The HiAP approach has also influenced the healthcare system, and the purpose of the healthcare system changes since the 1970s has been to increase quality and efficiency through better coordination and more collaboration. A wide range of complex care coordination initiatives have been developed. However, the results of their effects on clinically relevant patient benefits have been difficult to determine (Peterson et al., 2019: 90; Kersting, Kneer & Barzel, 2020). Still, multi-actor collaboration is critical to the successful implementation of public health services, but the health sector has gained little interest when promoting collaboration with sectors outside the health sector. This lack of attention may be regarded as a reaction to the *health imperialism* when the health sector overemphasizing public health as an intersectoral policy goal (Kriegner et al., 2020). However, during the past decades, public health and healthcare has taken up ideas about capacity building and empowerment. This means that a bottom-up approach supplements the top-down approach that dominated in the past, and a transition from public management (government) to co-management where many actors are equal partners in network organizations (governance).

According to HiAP approach, the primary healthcare, health promotion and community development shall be integrated into community health practice and become an approach to healthcare that involves enhancing community competence and creating community changes and development. However, according to Laverack and Labonte (2000: 261), public health services (such as health education and primary care services) in community-based settings have traditionally focused changes related to disease risks or unhealthy lifestyles on the deficiencies of individuals, the treatment of sick individuals and problem-solving by outside experts. This practice undermines clients' sense of capacity and self-worth, decreases their involvement in health-related decision-making, limits the use of community resources and weakens community ties. The empowerment discourse of health promoters as legitimized by the Ottawa Charter has created major tension in health promotion today. Many health promoters continue to exert power over the community through top-down programmes, while simultaneously inviting people to participate in emancipatory bottom-up processes, and they do not have a clear understanding of how community empowerment can be accommodated within health promotion programmes. Two seemingly different health promotion discourses coexist and have evolved into two distinct and somewhat exclusive approaches that are problematic to combine in practice (Laverack & Labonte, 2000: 256):

- The *conventional discourse* emphasizes top-down disease prevention through lifestyle management and vector control.
- The *communicative discourse* emphasizes social justice through bottom-up community empowerment, advocacy and partnership.

Cairney (2022) and Cairney, Denny and Mitchell (2022) write that these discourses are also present in public health research. For the most part, HiAP studies still treat policymaking as an instrumental technical exercise to find the right language to define the problems, solutions that work and the right model for intersectoral action and implementation. They, too, often ignore the fact that HiAP in practice is a communicative policymaking process where there are dilemmas and power conflicts between the actors involved. Godziewski (2020: 2) adds that, so far, research on HiAP has focused on technical implementation and less on the political challenges HiAP faces. These two discourses also exist in planning, and Sager (1990) calls them the concepts of calculation and communication. In our interpretation of HiAP, the great challenge is how to combine the conventional and instrumental discourse with the communicative discourse in the practice of planning, participation, partnership and policymaking. How to do this seems to be more developed in planning sciences than public health sciences.

The planning challenge – modernization versus mobilization

Instrumental rationality points towards the gains that the society can show through economy and science and has formed the foundation for understanding modernizing as an expression of progress and that progress is associated with better efficiency and rationalizing. However, scientists argue that Western societies suffer under the instrumental rationality and the neglect of communicative rationality and collective process and that the situation in general is a consequence of the modernization process in our societies (Habermas, 1996; Giddens, 1990). Dryzek (1990) blames the instrumental rationality for many of the crisis in the world and argues that the cure is communicative rationality and discursive democracy with participatory democracy, communicative action and practical reasoning.

If one uses the instrumental rationality as a foundation for reforms in the "modern state", the state shall become a more efficient instrument to produce output and outcome. But many scientists argue that this is not enough to legitimate the modern state. In addition, one must raise the moral question to what extent the state has become more democratic, just and humane. Eriksen (1993) substantiates this by asking if there is done enough to ensure that every group and their needs, interests and demands for respect are being looked after and to what extent the public sector activities are in accordance with valid moral and the standard court justice. He finds great shortages in today's presumption of modernizing, and he argues strongly for strengthen these normative values which can only be achieved through communicative rationality and mobilized citizens. A mobilized collective counterforce can be regarded as an individual and community capacity building process, a process based on the principle of empowerment with a balance between top-down support and external forces, and bottom-up support and mobilizing endogen resources.

In planning practice, one tries to meet these challenges caused by modernization by combining to different theoretical concepts: theory of rationality and theory of structuration. Both theories deal with how one perceives the situation and how one can understand and explain actors intended and performed actions.

- The *theory of rationality* makes a distinction and a dichotomy between the instrumental and a communicative rationality of how knowledge is connected to action, either through the exercise of power or through opinion formation. The work of Habermas is central, and he maintains that in practice, instrumental and communicative rationality are always combined (Habermas, 1996).

- The *theory of structuration* makes a distinction and a dichotomy between powerful actor's will-controlled actions (voluntaristic) and the structural influence from laws, regulations, norms, institutions, etc. (deterministic). The works of Giddens are central, and he maintains that both structure and agency play a role in shaping behaviour. Individuals shape and are shaped by social structures (Giddens, 1984; 1990).

The combination of the theoretical concepts involves a strengthening of the *horizontal power structure* through activating the civil society, the elected representatives and private businesses in collaborative processes. In this way, horizontal political power can be organized to supplement and oppose the sector dominated and *vertical power structure*. Many researchers agree upon this point of view and see the local community with a strong civil society and a strong democratic process as the main key to empower local and regional communities; see among others Forester (1993) and Storper (1997).

From this perspective, it becomes logical to empower local and regional communities to oppose the dominating vertical and mainly instrumental power structure (Friedmann & Weaver, 1979). Seen in relation to planning, this will involve strengthening planning's territorial dimension at the expense of the sector dimension. To put it another way, cross-sector collaboration can only be achieved by creating a territorial counterforce to the vertical and sector-based government structural forces. In a local and regional policy context and in public health work, this means that the bottom-up and mainly communicative power can equalize the top-down and mainly instrumental power and thus contribute to building of adequate local and regional development institutions (see Figure 1.1).

Case studies seem to show that integrated public health programmes with synergy between anti-poverty strategies, NGO and government collaboration, community participation, are probably most effective in improving health and development outcomes (Health Evidence Network, 2006: 15). Empowerment cannot be given to people or done to people but must come from processes where people empower themselves.

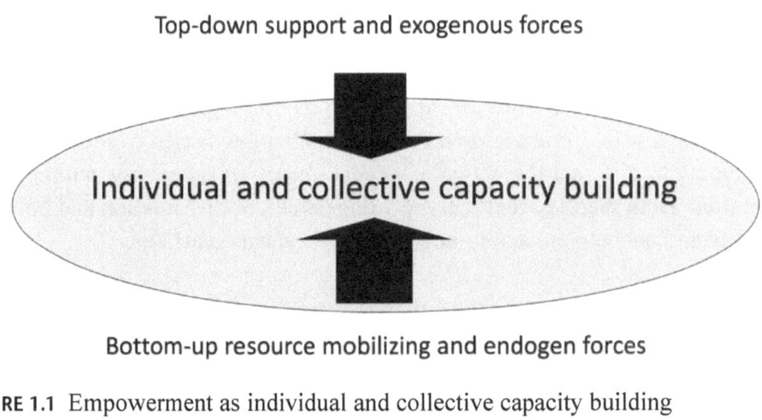

FIGURE 1.1 Empowerment as individual and collective capacity building

Sources: Based on Amdam (2010: 16).

External change agents may catalyse actions or help create arenas for people to learn, but empowerment occurs only if people create their own momentum, gains their own skills and advocates their own changes. Local, state and national government, as major players in the opportunity structure, must have a focus on empowerment strategies that force improved responsiveness to constituents, enhance transparency, uncorrupted government, greater efficiency and more equitable distribution of resources and services to communities (Health Evidence Network, 2006: 19).

The collaborative planning challenge – the pragmatic approach

There are many definitions of the word planning and many understandings of what planning amounts to (Alexander, 1984; 2016; 2000). Our understanding is similar to Friedmann's (1987: 39), when he describes planning as attempting to link scientific and technical knowledge to action in the public domain. However, this knowledge-action definition inhabits different approaches to public health planning and other forms of planning based on which theories are used when one argues to justify one's action. In academic discussions, instrumental and communicative planning are often viewed as being in opposition to each other, and researchers argue against each other based on artificially constructed and often mistaken views of what the two forms of planning truly involve. The result is often that they talk past each other, and that the development of theory and method halts. The same can be said about the actor versus structure approach to planning.

Collaborative planning can be regarded as a pragmatic attempt to handle both the instrumental versus communicative rationality dichotomy and the actor versus structure dichotomy (Alexander, 1984; Innes & Booher, 2002; 2015). Collaborative planning can be defined as a democratic process in which two or more actors who are mutually dependent on each other enter a constructive collaboration to define problems and find solutions since the actors are different but can enter into intermediate agreements and coexist simultaneously as they can agree to disagree (Healey, 1997; Healey, 2009). The purpose is to involve people in discourses that can transform the communicative power into new actions and political power with the legitimacy to implement needed structural change. The planner in collaborative processes thus becomes one of many actors contributing to the process both as expert with knowledge and as facilitator of the process.

Responding effectively to public health situations in society today requires collective action, and collective action requires both meaningful health planning and an understanding of society's resources (Salem, 2005: 379). Public health planning has evolved over the course of half a century from the problem/programme-focused planning of its earliest stages into more comprehensive approaches and then into the strategic planning of today (Lenihan, 2005). By use of the approach *Mobilizing for Action through Planning and Partnership* (MAPP), public health planning has evolved from the more traditional needs assessment and programme planning approaches, typically addressing single issues, to a model that is grounded in strategic planning concepts that tries to put the most important issues on the agenda and to include new and diverse partners in the process. However, the strategic approach to planning, which comes from the private sector, cannot be easily applied to the public sector (Bryson & Roering, 1987). Closely related to the strategic approach is the dynamic systemic thinking including feedback processes and learning environment (Corso, Wiesner & Lenihan, 2005: 388).

Many of the planning models that are used the most in public health planning practice are dominated by a top-down programme implementation approach and regard planning as a linear process (McKenzie, Neiger & Smeltzer, 2005). Wilson (2004: 409) therefore argues that national health programmes need to be structured such that the advantages of local and regional approaches to public health challenges are balanced against the benefits of a coordinated central response and that policymakers need to address the unique challenges of public health governance (McKenzie, Neiger & Smeltzer, 2005). A collaboration between instrumental top-down and communicative bottom-up politics are needed to support HiAP with necessary capacity and legitimacy. According to instrumental rationality, HiAP can be legitimized by technical and economic efficiency and cost/benefit accounting. Communicative rationality, on the other hand, can help provide plans and institutions with the kind of meaningfulness that relates to the public sector's purpose of being sustainable, democratic, transparent, fair and humane. Therefore, collaborative planning with the combination of top-down and bottom-up politics can become best practice for the implementation of HiAP approaches (Cain et al., 2022). However, we will add that active citizens are a prerequisite to succeed.

The participation challenge – collecting knowledge or building competence

According to the Health Evidence Network (2006: 8), participation is seen as a complex and interactive process, which can grove or diminish based on the unfolding of power relations. Participation can make up the base of empowerment in public health but is alone insufficient if the process does not build a capacity for further community actions. Participation is critical in reducing the dependency on health professionals and ensuring cultural and local sensitivity of programmes, but participation is not predictable in its outcomes and happens with or without professionals. Therefore, professionals' role in community development process must shift from dominant expert in top-down politics to supportive or facilitative process manager in collaborative policymaking.

Bryson et al. (2013) write that there are many purposes for public participation in planning like advancing democracy, social justice, learning and the quality of plans, and public participation processes are sometimes oriented to small groups of key stakeholders, sometimes to interested public and sometimes to the public general. Participation in planning emerged in the 1960s and has now become a part of the *communicative and collaborative turn* in planning (Healey, 1993).

Broad participation in planning and development processes is now regarded a necessity to achieve empowerment in communities. However, there is research that shows that participation in regional and local planning and partnerships tends to become a professional elite activity involving employees from public and private sectors rather than citizens and stakeholders (Swyngedouw, 2005). Many planners and researchers have experienced that even comprehensive participation does not necessarily challenge the established political power if those in power can choose to consider all the views expressed. Many planners have also experienced that consulting is widely used in planning and development processes both in organizations and communities to legitimize decisions that are already made.

In the instrumental planning, the capacity to act is often taken for granted as long as the work can be legitimized by law and regulations and that the benefit of the work is greater than the cost. The process is linear, and the planner is an expert who, based on collected knowledge, produces a professionally sound plan, which the client or others must adopt and then implement. Participation is often limited, and the purpose of participation is often the acquisition of knowledge to make the plan good so that the implementation meets the least possible resistance. In theory, such instrumental planning can be carried out if one has full knowledge of the situation, clear goals and a great deal of control over means in the form of command power over desired and necessary actions. This form of planning characterizes top-down politics. But this is a different form of planning than the one need in collaborative processes in communities and organizations. The starting point here is a critique of the instrumental planning that turns planning into a professional activity that creates dependency between the planner as expert and plan-maker, and the client as plan-implementer. In collaborative planning, it is the planner's role to create a learning process that obliges the participants to carry out their part of the plan. The purpose of participation in such planning is to contribute to individual competence and collective capacity building so that as many people as possible accept the plan and participate in its implementation (Amdam, 2018; 2020). Collaborative planning therefore emphasizes strengthening legitimacy through dialogues about the situation, the future and the methods of action so that the participants' capacity to act is based on an acknowledgement of what is important to have on the agenda and how they can act to achieve the desired result.

Lane (2005) has published a clear overview of participation in planning related to various approaches and theories that have dominated for periods. The starting point is Arnstein's (1969) *Ladder of Citizen Participation*, which was developed as a criticism of a federal (United States) urban planning programme. Arnstein writes a general statement that still may be actual: "There is a critical difference between going through the empty ritual of participation and having the real power needed to affect the outcome of the process" (Arnstein, 1969: 217). Arnstein's ladder model has eight steps. The lowest step is the manipulation of the inhabitants, then therapy, information, consultation, placation, partnership, delegated and citizen control.

This ladder has undoubtedly had a great impact on the public participation practice in planning, and the original and variants of it can be found both in textbooks and in official planning guides. But the ladder has also faced criticism and mainly because of two circumstances (Painter, 1992: 23–24). First, the ladder does not distinguish between potential and real power. Participating at different levels in the ladder entails a formal and potential power for participation and involvement in the planning, but it is only when one sees the results of the plan that one can see who had real and perhaps also informal power in the process. Second, the ladder is criticized for a naïve understanding of planning and policymaking as an instrumental and linear process with a single decision at the end of the process. In this way, the ladder-model neglects that the process has many stages underway where actors with power can influence the design of the process, the agenda, the collection and analysis of data, the definition of problems and solutions, the legitimization through formal decisions, and the implementation and evaluation of the results.

Overall, the ladder can function as a knowledge gettering process with the aim to enlighten the situation and improve the decisions, but the decisions makers are in a position to prioritize what knowledge and arguments they will give most weight. Participation thus mainly becomes an instrument for asking residents for input that later can be filtered by people in power to underpin the plans and the decisions. For HiAP, the danger with this approach is that participation in planning may be used as a tool to collect information so that public health workers and the health sector can create what they perceive as good public health plans.

In our opinion, a real alternative to the ladder of citizen participation must place the citizen at the centre and function as a collaborative empowerment process (Hyung Hur, 2006) and this model should, in our opinion, be called the *spiral of citizen participation* (Amdam, 2018; Amdam, 2020). Friedmann (1978) contributes to this understanding of empowerment with the social practice epistemology in which the individual and collective action capacity emerges in a critical reflection process that alternates between radial practice and critical reflection (see Chapter 2). This empowerment process requires that actors from the public, private and voluntary sectors collaborate as equal actors to set the agenda, design solutions, implement actions and discuss experiences in a continuous spiral-like process that contributed to increased power and capacity (Healey, 2003; Healey, 2009).

Davoudi (2015) argues likewise, and she sums up the planning debate by emphasizing that in collaborative processes, planning should shift the focus away from instrumental evidence-based knowledge because such knowledge has limited value in planning as an activity. Based on a pragmatic theoretical perspective, Davoudi (2015) therefore argues that instead of focusing on the term objective and evidence-based knowledge in planning, rather turn attention to the term knowing and to assume that *collaborative planning is a practice in knowing*. She writes that instead of considering the truth as something that planners have (or seek to obtain), one should focus on the practice of knowing as something that planners do. Instead of thinking that knowledge has an instrumental place in the planning process, it is more useful to think of planning as a process of recognition and learning (Davoudi, 2015: 317). She describes planning as a critical reflective learning process where the actors should show practical judgement (prudence/wisdom) towards each other when they discuss the central elements in planning. Therefore, participants in collaborative planning should exercise wisdom (phronesis) as practical judgement based on a critical reflective process that combines *knowing why* (moral choices), *knowing what* (theories and concepts), *knowing how* (crafts and skills) and *doing* (actions) (Davoudi, 2015: 321).

Another good professional word for practical judgement in such processes is *collaborative competence*, which is precisely about being able to do something together with others. The elements in the term competence are values, knowledge, skills and actions (Amdam, 2020; Lai, 2021). Competence differs from knowledge in that it is not suitable for being stored. Competence is something one develop over time and which enables one to consider situations, needs, goals and other actors. Competence is something that one has as individuals (individual be able to) but which can be further developed and strengthened in interaction with other people. When a community collaborate about doing and to answer the questions why, what and how to proceed, the community strengthen the capacity to act (collectively be able to).

The partnership challenge – governance in shadow of government

Rhodes (1997) writes that while government refers to a political system based on well-defined hierarchical relationships linked to a national and elected governing body, governance refers to a looser structure with fragmented political and economic power where the boundaries between and within the private, public and voluntary sectors are erased. Governance implies the creation of new structures that is a result of the interaction of different actors.

In political theory, the term *government* refers to the formal institutions of the state and their monopoly of legitimate coercive power. Government is the formal institutional structure and location of authoritative decision-making in the modern state, like ministries, agencies, municipalities and counties. The concept of governance, in contrast, is wider and directs attention to the distribution of power both internally and externally to the state. Governance is about governmental and non-governmental network organizations working together in a new planning and implementing structure based on partnership between public, private and voluntary sector and between national, regional and local level. In practice, such multi-actor collaboration lives in the shadow of the formal government structure (Héritier & Lehmkuhl, 2008).

Partnership is a common term for network organizations and multi-actor collaboration, and partnership is defined as a binding collaboration between sovereign parties in a pre-negotiated community of interests (Rhodes, 1997). Based on

Torfing (2016), partnerships in the form of collaborative network processes can be referred to as processes where two or more actors (from the public, private or voluntary sector) form a constructive collaboration to define a problem and find solutions based on that fact that they function as different actors but who can set up agreements and coexist while having disagreements.

Stoker (1998: 22) expresses that recognizing the power dependence in collective actions implies accepting that intentions do not always match outcomes because network organizations are based on interdependency, trust and mutual interest of achieving outcome they cannot create alone. However, the potential outcome from the partnership will always be compared with the transaction coast of staying in contact with the partners. The basic question for the participants seems to be *what is in it for me* as a partner. Thus, the governance and partnerships' capacity to solve problems is strongly dependent on the acceptance and legitimacy of the network organization.

In local and regional planning and development, there has been an obvious turn from sectorized government to partnerships and governance. As far as we can see, the same turning process is going on in public health (Vega & Irwin, 2004; Haines, Kuruvilla & Borchert, 2004). The intention is seemingly to supplement the traditional government structure in public health with a governance structure with partnerships. Partnership as a tool in public health practice is built upon a long history of various types of local public health collaboration who work in teams towards a set of shared public health goals. It has been documented that if these partnerships function as they should, they promote health across sectors and professions, and between public, private and voluntary institutions, at a collective level and they change behaviour at the individual level (Gillies, 1998), and it is documented that wicked, uncontrollable and stubborn problems are handled most successfully when local health management manages to establish partnerships that combine democratic legitimacy with institutional action capacity (Moon, 2020). Therefore, there is a strong need for cross-sector networking and for public sector managers to take part in partnerships and collaborative local and regional planning and development. Governance institutions in the form of network organizations and partnerships must be established and maintained in collaborative political processes (Jessop, 1997). However, such successful partnerships are difficult to achieve (Axelsson & Axelsson, 2006; Héritier & Lehmkuhl, 2008).

The policy process challenge – having political capacity and legitimacy

The policy process can be viewed in a system-theoretical perspective. The systemic approach to policymaking processes is well known from different authors and has been developed since Easton (1965) was one of the first who used it. In the simplest form, the system model has input, throughput and output elements and feedback loops from the output to the input element.

Internationally, a lot of research are published on collaborative policy processes and on associated forms of governance and they maintain that successful partnerships require that they have institutional capacity for action and that the power they exercise has democratic legitimacy (Osborne, 2009; Sørensen & Torfing, 2009; Bryson, Crosby & Bloomberg, 2014). In addition, it is documented that the partnerships' legitimacy and the capacity to act are mutually dependent on each other (Christensen, Lægreid & Rykkja, 2016; Christensen & Lægreid, 2020), that is, without capacity for action, no legitimacy and without legitimacy, no capacity for action (see Chapter 5).

Democratic legitimacy refers to the legitimacy that is created by the fact that the process and the results reflect the will of the people (Rosanvallon, 2018). This will can incorporate general values related to ideal state and an ideal society with central values such as democracy, local and global sustainable development, self-government, freedom of expression, equality, justice and social benefit. This form of legitimacy is by Scott (2014) called *regulatory legitimacy* which expressed in laws, rules and regulations. Other forms are *normative legitimacy* which expresses what is perceived as important in society, *cognitive legitimacy* that are mental representations that make up the nature of social reality and *pragmatic legitimacy* which is linked to the production of goods and services and their utility compared to costs.

Having political capacity to act can be interpreted as having political power. Lukes (1974) has made a fundamental statement on this topic, and he distinguishes between three dimensions in the execution of power. Actors in this context can be individuals, groups, organizations and political institutions, and they can act both intentionally and unintentionally. The *one-dimensional* form of execution of power represents an operative form of power where one actor has the power to control another actor's actions, i.e. the output-side. The *two-dimensional* power comes in the form having the power to make decisions that can solve the problem. In a policy process model, this power is expressed through having control over the decision-making activity, and it can also be called control over the throughput side of the policy process. The *three-dimensional* power represents control over the political agenda. In relation to a policymaking model, this involves having control of the input side and the influence on for instance what people think and care about and how strongly people argue their case. In addition, the *four-dimensional* power being able to decide the design of the policy process, including progress, content, and participants, secures the existence of political institution.

Compared to the simplest form of the system model, Pollitt and Bouckaert (2000) have a more elaborated contribution to the systemic approach, and their model puts focus on important political and public issues (see Figure 1.2).

Figure 1.2 conveys that based on the outcomes and impacts of previous policies, needs emerge and goals are formulated for changes, which through the process, are concretized as goals, and put on the political agenda (input side and three-dimensional power). Then follows what can be called a problem-solving and

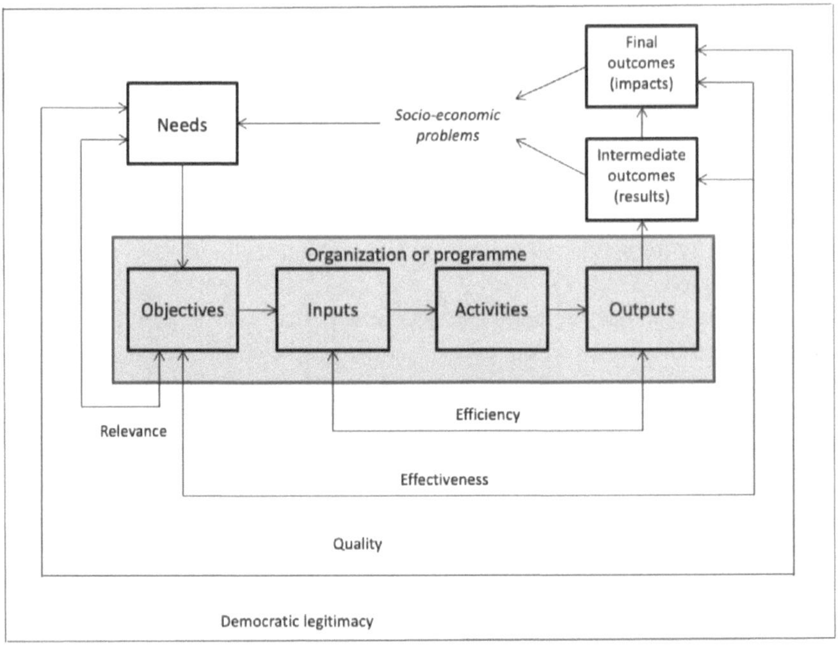

FIGURE 1.2 The policy process

Source: Based on Pollitt and Bouckaert (2000: 106) and Amdam (2010: 8).

decision-making production (throughput side and two-dimensional power), which then entails concrete activities, products, achievements and effects (output side and one-dimensional power). What one should notice is that the model makes a clear distinction between activities/product/achievements (output) and the results/consequences/effects of these (outcome/impacts). One reason for this is that results in the form of outcomes and impacts are more difficult to measure than activities, products and achievements (outputs). In addition, it is also more difficult to document logical connections between the production (inputs) and the results (outcomes) than between the production (input) and the activities (outputs). This is because there are so many other factors that come into play. This situation creates an accountability deficit with problems keeping the actors and institutions accountable for the lack of outcome and impacts. For example, the public sector can easily account for its production in terms of activities, but the sector faces problems when the sector must account for the results of production in terms of what the production has meant for the citizens and to what extent there are other conditions that have meant something for the result.

The complexity of this model clarifies the need for designing the process (the four-dimensional power) and to secure that a collaborative process included HiAP can only be regarded as successful if the process contributes to increased efficiency, effectiveness, quality and legitimacy.

HiAP must contribute to increased production and efficiency (outputs)

The term *efficiency* is linked to the input and output sides and says something about how much resources the process uses to produce certain products and achievements. This is also called cost-effective and can be summed up in the question of whether one produces in the right way. For HiAP, one of the critical questions is whether the public health work practice is according to established standards and routines is organized in a cost-effective way and that the work provides necessary and desired activities/actions.

HiAP must contribute to increased effectiveness (outcomes/results)

The concept of *effectiveness* is often specified as goal-effective to emphasize that it is about the extent to which the process's products and achievements produce the desired results and effects in relation to formulated concrete objectives/goals. This means whether one produces what is considered the right in relation to the current objectives. For HiAP, this may mean that the public health is reaching its specific and quantifiable goals like how many patients shall be treated in a month, how many shall be on the waiting list at the end of a month, how many have got vaccines, etc.

HiAP must contribute to increased quality (outcomes/impacts)

In addition, there are the long-term consequences of the production, the extent to which the production affects satisfying the needs in the society (*quality*) and can be called need-effective. These results are difficult to measure, and it is often difficult to document connections between cause and effect. But results in terms of measured quality are in no way less important than results in relation to measured efficiency and effectiveness. If we stick to the example from the health sector, a high degree of quality imply that the needs of the clients and citizens are met to their satisfaction.

HiAP must contribute to increased democratic legitimacy

Democratic legitimacy can come from above by superior governing powers by law establish institution, issuing they orders and purposes, delegating power to them, granting they money, etc. (input legitimacy). Legitimacy from below comes from the people and from how strongly they support the sector or topic (output/outcome legitimacy). Democratic legitimacy thus concerns the extent to which policy processes can produce cost-effective and lasting solutions to problems that are in line with people's interests, needs and the generally accepted fundamental societal and public sector values (value-effective). Low democratic legitimacy implies that an institution does not fulfil its purpose and satisfy public values. This situation can threaten its existence and for the public health sector, low democratic legitimacy can imply discussion about privatization of services, for example, the specialist health services.

In this legitimating process, instrumental rationality is necessary but not sufficient. According to Banfield (1973), it can ideally be expected from instrumental processes that inputs, outputs and outcome measurements are based on causal relationships and on the maximization of stakeholders' benefit. In many areas of society, it is difficult to demonstrate the connections between cause and effect and often no evidence-based knowledge exists. The reason for this is that people interpret situations differently and that they have different needs, interests and values, which means that actions that are logical to some can be seen as illogical by others and that both knowledge and logic becomes subjective and dependent on time and space. Hence, actors following the same procedure can achieve different outputs and outcomes and a method that is successful in one context cannot be copied to a different context.

This does not imply that in situations where one lacks evidence-based knowledge that *determines the actions* and where the implementation of the plan is dependent on many actors, one is left without planning and leadership tools. It is in such situations that the combination of instrumental and communicative rationality in collaborative processes is best suited. In the absence of an actor with the power to make plans and implement, the alternative is to start planning processes where the actors can gather broad knowledge about the problem and make proposed solutions that are meaningful to them. In this situation, scientific knowledge can *inform the practice*. The purpose of the planning process is thus changed from a having power to make and implement a plan as a *product* to a planning process creating power in opinion and will formation process with emphasis on broad participation and extensive learning. Thus, planning and implementation become one and the same process and the actors' collaboration is made legitimate through the democratic process itself (Amdam, 1997; Amdam, 2001; Amdam, 2020). Accordingly, the planner's role changes from being the expert who *gives answers* to becoming the process-leader who *asks questions* to stimulate reflection among the participants in the process.

Conclusion

The concept of HiAP has evolved over time with the World Health Organization as a driving force. The approach emphasizes planning, participation, partnership and making politic with institutional capacity and democratic legitimacy. But the dilemma for HiAP and other multi-actor collaborations is that without capacity, they have no legitimacy, and without legitimacy, they have no capacity. In practice, the HiAP is facing two main challenges: how to balance the instrumental and communicative rationality, and how to balance the relation between actors and structures. We find that the challenges are discussed in HiAP and in healthcare, but in planning theory, the needed combination is more developed in the form of collaborative planning. Collaborative planning can transform local and regional communicative power to oppose the dominant instrumental sectorized national power and thus creates new politics and political institutions. Hence, HiAP, as a collaborative process, must deliver increased efficiency, effectiveness, quality and legitimacy to gain more institutional capacity and democratic legitimacy for HiAP.

When summing up the discussion in this chapter, we find that HiAP needs a better balance between instrumental and communicative rationality, but how we govern our society makes structural forces which can stimulate or hamper the balance. There is a need for discussing how the challenges we have presented in this chapter have been handled under different planning thoughts and policy traditions and their impact on HiAP, which is the topic in the next chapter.

The structure of the book

Our main message in this book is that HiAP needs to be practised as radical New Public Governance and the argumentation goes like this: In Chapter 1, we have clarified the term *HiAP* and claimed that HiAP is a multi-actor collaboration about policymaking using planning and partnerships as tools. HiAP represents what we call governance, which is dependent on the formal government's willingness to participate and support. In Chapter 2, we discuss different governing system and their ability to make HiAP successful and we argue that the radical New Public Governance is best suited. This governing system is a reaction to the fragmentation, silo-thinking and unit-egoism that characterize the other governing systems and has the purpose to legitimacy political changes and establish more collaborative process between involved institutions and actors. In Chapter 3, we discuss how Habermas' political will formation process can be adapted to collaborative planning and become a process supporting HiAP with the needed institutional capacity and democratic legitimacy to succeed. In Chapter 4, we substantiate this will formation process in the ISTOL-planning model with relations between the development variables: context, mobilization, organizing and implementation, and planning tools: institutional, strategic, tactical and operative planning, and in Chapter 5, we discuss how this model can be utilized in monitoring and managing the HiAP, as a planning process, using the different planning tools to maintain and increase the different forms of democratic legitimacy and institutional capacity. These relations are illustrated with the planning staircase. In Chapter 6, we use the planning staircase do discuss the democratic legitimacy and institutional capacity of HiAP in three cases. The cases are promoting public health in the Baltic Sea Region (HEPRO), HiAP in Norway before the COVID-19 pandemic and HiAP in Møre and Romsdal County before and during the pandemic.

References

Alexander, E. R. 1984. After rationality, what? A review of responses to paradigm breakdown. *Journal of the American Planning Association*, Winter 1984: 62–69. https://doi.org/10.1080/01944368408976582

Alexander, E. R. 2000. Rationality revisited: Planning paradigms in a post-postmodernist perspective. *Journal of Planning Education and Research*, 19: 242–256. https://doi.org/10.1177/0739456x0001900303

Alexander, E. R. 2016. There is no planning – Only planning practices: Notes for spatial planning theories. *Planning Theory*, 15 (1): 91–103. https://www.jstor.org/stable/26098733

Amdam, R. 1997. Empowerment planning in local communities. *International Planning Studies*, 2 (3): 329–345. http://dx.doi.org/10.1080/13563479708721688

Amdam, R. 2001. Empowering new regional political institutions – A Norwegian case. *Journal of Planning Theory & Practice*, 2 (2): 169–185. https://doi.org/10.1080/14649350120068786

Amdam, R. 2018. Samarbeidsdriven planlegging. In: Aarsæther, N., Falleth, E., Nyseth, T. & Kristiansen, R. (eds.) *Plan og samfunn: System, praksis, teori*. Oslo: Cappelen Damm Akademisk.

Amdam, R. 2020. Planning and innovation in a collaborative framework. In: Hagen, A. & Higdem, U. (eds.) *Innovation in Public Planning. Calculate, Communicate and Innovate*. Cham, Switzerland: Palgrave Macmillan.

Amdam, R. 2023. "Health in all policies" in Norwegian municipalities—Dilemmas and lack of legitimacy and capacity. *International Journal of Health Planning and Management*, 38: 1345–1359. http://dx.doi.org/10.1002/hpm.3664

Arnstein, S. R. 1969. A ladder of citizen participation. *Journal of the American Institute of Planners*, 35 (4): 216–224. https://doi.org/10.1080/01944366908977225

Axelsson, R. & Axelsson, S. B. 2006. Integration and collaboration in public health—A conceptual framework. *The International Journal of Health Planning and Management*, 21 (1): 75–88. https://doi.org/10.1002/hpm.826

Banfield, E. C. 1973. Ends and means in planning. In: Faludi, A. (ed.) *A Reader in Planning Theory*. Oxford: Pergamon Press.

Bryson, J. M., Crosby, B. C. & Bloomberg, L. 2014. Public value governance: Moving beyond traditional public administration and new public management. *Public Administration Review*, 74 (4): 445–456. https://doi.org/10.1111/puar.12238

Bryson, J. M., Quick, K. S., Slotterback, C. S. & Crosby, B. C. 2013. Designing public participation processes. *Public Administration Review*, 73 (1): 23–34. http://www.jstor.org/stable/23355431

Bryson, J. M. & Roering, W. D. 1987. Applying private-sector strategic planning in the public sector. *Journal of the American Planning Association*, 53 (1): 9–22. https://doi.org/10.1080/01944368708976631

Cain, R. et al. 2022. Improving health across sectors: Best Practices for the implementation of health in all policies approaches. *Preventive Medicine Reports*, 29 (2022):101961 https://doi.org/10.1016/j.pmedr.2022.101961

Cairney, P. 2022. Understanding public policy. In: *Theories and Issues*. London: Bloomsbury Academic.

Cairney, P., Denny, E. S. & Mitchell, H. 2022. How can policy theory help to address the expectations gap in preventive public health and 'Health in all Policies'? In: Fafard, P., Cassola, A., & de Leeuw, E. (eds.) *Integrating Science and Politics for Public Health*: 239–265. Cham, Switzerland: Palgrave Macmillan.

Castro, E. M., Van Regenmortel, T., Vanhaecht, K., Sermeus, W. & Van Hecke, A. 2016. Patient empowerment, patient participation and patient-centeredness in hospital care: A concept analysis based on a literature review. *Patient Education and Counseling*, 99 (12): 1923–1939. https://doi.org/10.1016/j.pec.2016.07.026

Christensen, T. & Lægreid, P. 2020. Balancing governance capacity and legitimacy: How the Norwegian government handled the COVID-19 crisis as a high performer. *Public Administration Review*, 80 (5): 774–779. https://doi.org/10.1111/puar.13241
Christensen, T., Lægreid, P. & Rykkja, L. H. 2016. Organizing for crisis management: Building governance capacity and legitimacy. *Public Administration Review*, 76 (6): 887–897. https://doi.org/10.1111/puar.12558
Corso, L. C., Wiesner, P. J. & Lenihan, P. 2005. Developing the MAPP community health improvement tool. *Public Health Management Practice*, 11 (5): 387–392. https://doi.org/10.1097/00124784-200509000-00003
Davoudi, S. 2015. Planning as practice of knowing. *Planning Theory*, 14 (3): 316–331. https://doi.org/10.1177/1473095215575919
Dryzek, J. S. 1990. *Discursive Democracy. Politics, Policy, and Political Science*. Cambridge: Cambridge University Press.
Easton, S. 1965. *A System Analysis of Political Life*. New York, NY: Wiley.
Eriksen, E. O. 1993. *Den offentlige dimensjonen. Verdier og styring i offentlig sektor*. Tromsø/Bergen: Tano Aschehoug.
Forester, J. 1993. *Critical Theory, Public Policy and Planning Practice: Toward a Critical Pragmatism*. Albany, NY: University of New York Press.
Friedmann, J. 1978. The epistemology of social practice: A critique of objective knowledge. *Theory and Society*, 6: 75–92. https://doi.org/10.1007/bf01566158
Friedmann, J. 1987. *Planning in the Public Domain. From Knowledge to Action*. Princeton, NJ: Princeton University Press.
Friedmann, J. & Weaver, C. 1979. *Territory and Function. The Evolution of Regional Planning*. London: Edward Arnold.
Giddens, A. 1984. *The Constitutions of Society: Outline of the Theory of Structuration*. Berkeley, CA: University of California Press.
Giddens, A. 1990. *The Consequences of Modernity*. Stanford, CA: Stanford University Press.
Gillies, P. 1998. Effectiveness of alliances and partnerships in health promotion. *Health Promotion International*, 13 (2): 99–120. https://doi.org/10.1093/heapro/13.2.99
Godziewski, C. 2020. Evidence and power in EU governance of health promotion: Discursive obstacles to a "Health in all policies" approach. *Journal of Common Market Studies*, 58 (5): 1307–1324. https://doi.org/10.1111/jcms.13042
Guglielmin, M., Muntaner, C., O'Campo, P. & Shankardass, K. 2018. A scoping review of the implementation of health in all policies at the local level. *Health Policy*, 122 (3): 284–292. https://doi.org/10.1016/j.healthpol.2017.12.005
Habermas, J. 1996. *Between Facts and Norms: Contributions to a Discourse Theory of Law and Democracy*. Cambridge, MA: MIT Press.
Haines, A., Kuruvilla, S. & Borchert, M. 2004. Bridging the implementation gap between knowledge and action for health. *Bulletin of the World Health Organization*, 82 (10): 724–731. https://iris.who.int/handle/10665/269259
Healey, P. 1993. Planning through debate: The communicative turn in planning theory. In: Fischer, F. & Forester, J. (eds.) *The Argumentative Turn in Policy Analysis and Planning*. Durham and London: Duke University Press.
Healey, P. 1997. *Collaborative Planning. Shaping Places in Fragmented Societies*. London: Macmillan Press.
Healey, P. 2003. Collaborative planning in perspective. *Planning Theory*, 2 (2): 101–123. https://doi.org/10.1177/14730952030022002
Healey, P. 2009. The pragmatic tradition in planning thought. *Journal of Planning Education and Research*, 28 (3): 277–292. https://doi.org/10.1177/0739456x08325175
Health Evidence Network (HEN). 2006. *What Is the Evidence on Effectiveness of Empowerment to Improve Health?* World Health Organization, Europe. Copenhagen: WHO Regional Office for Europe.

Héritier, A. & Lehmkuhl, D. 2008. Introduction: The shadow of hierarchy and new modes of governance. *Journal of Public Policy*, 28 (19): 1–17. http://dx.doi.org/10.1017/S0143814X08000755

Huang, C. L. & Wang, H. H. 2005. Community health development: What is it? *International Nursing Review*, 52 (1): 13–17. https://doi.org/10.1111/j.1466-7657.2004.00259.x

Hyung Hur, M. 2006. Empowerment in terms of theoretical perspectives: Exploring a typology of the process and components across disciplines. *Journal of Community Psychology*, 34 (5): 523–540. https://doi.org/10.1002/jcop.20113

Innes, J. E. & Booher, D. E. 2002. Network power in collaborative planning. *Journal of Planning Education and Research*, 21: 221–236. https://doi.org/10.1177/0739456x020210030

Innes, J. E. & Booher, D. E. 2015. A turning point for planning theory? Overcoming dividing discourses. *Planning Theory*, 14 (2): 195–213. https://doi.org/10.1177/1473095213519356

Jessop, B. 1997. A neo-Gramscian approach to the regulation of urban regimes: Accumulation strategies, hegemonic projects, and governance. In: Lauria, M. (ed.) *Reconstructing Urban Regime Theory: Regulating Urban Politics in a Global Economy*: 51–73. London: Sage.

Kersting, C., Kneer, M. & Barzel, A. 2020. *Patient-relevant outcomes: What are we talking about?* A scoping review to improve conceptual clarity. *BMC Health Service Research*, 20 (1). https://doi.org/10.1186/s12913-020-05442-9

Kickbusch, I. 2003. The contribution of the world health organization to a new public health and health promotion. *American Journal of Public Health*, 93 (3): 383–388. https://doi.org/10.2105/ajph.93.3.383

Kokko, S., Liveng, A. & Torp, S. 2018. 20 years of health promotion research in the Nordic countries: Health, wellbeing and physical activity. *Scandinavian Journal of Public Health*, 46 (20): 3–6. https://doi.org/10.1177/1403494817751041

Kriegner, S., Ottersen, T., Rottingen, J.-A. & Gopinathan, U. 2020. Promoting intersectoral collaboration through the evaluations of public health interventions: Insights from key informants in 6 European countries. *International Journal of Health Policy and Management*, 10 (2): 67–76. https://doi.org/10.34172/ijhpm.2020.19

Lai, L. 2021. *Strategisk kompetanseledelse*. Bergen: Fagbokforlaget.

Lane, M. B. 2005. Public participation in planning: An intellectual history. *Australian Geographer*, 36 (3): 283–299. https://doi.org/10.1080/00049180500325694

Laverack, G. & Labonte, R. 2000. A planning framework for community empowerment goals within health promotion. *Health Policy and Planning*, 15 (3): 255–262. https://doi.org/10.1093/heapol/15.3.255

Lenihan, P. 2005. MAPP and the evolution of planning in public health practice. *Public Health Management Practice*, 11 (5): 381–386. https://doi.org/10.1097/00124784-200509000-00002

Lukes, S. 1974. *Power: A Radical View*. London: Macmillan.

McKenzie, J. F., Neiger, B. L. & Smeltzer, J. L. 2005. *Planning, Implementation, and Evaluating Health Promotion Programs*. London: Pearson Education. Benjamin Cummings.

Moon, M. J. 2020. Fighting against COVID-19 with agility, transparency, and participation: Wicked policy problems and new governance challenges. *Public Administration Review*, 80 (4): 651–656. https://doi.org/10.1111/puar.13214

Osborne, S. P. 2009. *The New Public Governance? Emerging Perspectives on the Theory and Practice of Public Governance*. London: Routledge.

Painter, M. 1992. Participation and power. In: Munro-Clarke, M. (ed.) *Citizen Participation in Government*. Sydney: Hale and Ironmonger.

Peterson, K., Anderson, J. & Bourne, D. et al. 2019. Health care coordination theoretical frameworks: A systematic scoping review to increase their understanding and use in practice. *Journal of General Internal Medicine*, 34 (1): 90–98. https://doi.org/10.1007/s11606-019-04966-z

Pollitt, C. & Bouckaert, G. 2000. *Public Management Reform: A Comparative Analysis – New Public Management, Governance, and the Neo-Weberian State*. Oxford: Oxford University Press.

Rhodes, R. A. W. 1997. *Understanding Governance. Policy Networks, Governance, Reflexivity and Accountability*. Bristol; Philadelphia, PA: Open University Press.

Rittel, H. W. & Webber, M. A. 1973. Dilemmas in a general theory of planning. *Policy Sciences*, 4: 155–169. http://dx.doi.org/10.1007/BF01405730

Rosanvallon, P. 2018. *Good Government. Democracy Beyond Elections*. Cambridge, MA: Harvard University Press.

Rose, R. 1979. Ungovernability: Is there fire behind the smoke? *Political Studies*, 27 (3): 351–370. https://doi.org/10.1111/j.1467-9248.1979.tb01209.x

Sager, T. 1990. *Communicate or Calculate. Planning Theory and Social Science Concepts in a Contingency Perspective*. NORDPLAN Dissertation 11. Stockholm: Nordic Institute for Studies in Urban and Regional Planning.

Salem, E. 2005. The promise of MAPP: A transformational tool for public health practice. *Public Health Management Practice*, 11 (5): 379–380. https://doi.org/10.1097/00124784-200509000-00001

Schiefloe, P. M. 2021. The corona crisis: A wicked problem. *Scandinavian Journal of Public Health, 49* (1): 5–8. https://doi.org/10.1177/1403494820970767

Scott, W. R. 2014. *Institutions and Organizations: Ideas, Interests, and Identities. 4th* edition. London: Sage Publications.

Sørensen, E. & Torfing, J. 2009. Making governance networks effective and democratic through metagovernance. *Public Administration*, 87 (2): 234–258. https://doi.org/10.1111/j.1467-9299.2009.01753.x

Ståhl, T. 2018. Health in all policies: From rhetoric to implementation and evaluation – The Finnish experience. *Scandinavian Journal of Public Health*, 46 (20): 38–46. https://doi.org/10.1177/1403494817743895

Stoker, G. 1998. Governance as theory, five propositions. *Social Science Journal*, 50: 17–28. https://doi.org/10.1111/1468-2451.00106

Storper, M. 1997. *The Regional World. Territorial Development in a Global Economy*. New York, NY & London: Guilford Press.

Swyngedouw, E. 2005. Governance innovation and the citizen: The Janus face of governance-beyond-the-state. *Urban Studies*, 42 (11): 1191–2006. https://doi.org/10.1080/00420980500279869

Torfing, J. 2016. *Collaborative Innovation in Public Sector*. Washington, DC: Georgetown University Press.

Vega, J. & Irwin, A. 2004. Tackling health inequalities: New approaches in public policy. *Bulletin of the World Health Organization*, 82 (7): 482. https://iris.who.int/handle/10665/269187

Weber, M. 2020. From alma ata to the SDGs: The politics of global health governance and the elusive "health for all". *Global Governance: A Review of Multilateralism and International Organizations*, 26 (1): 176–197. https://doi.org/10.1163/19426720-02601005

Weber, E. P. & Khademian, A. M. 2008. Wicked problems, knowledge challenges, and collaborative capacity builders in network settings. *Public Administration Review*, 68 (2): 334–349. https://www.jstor.org/stable/25145606

Wilson, K. 2004. The complexities of multi-level governance in public health. *Canadian Journal of Public Health*, 95 (6): 409–412. https://doi.org/10.1007/bf03403981

Winslow, C.-E. A. 1920. The untilled fields of public health. *Modern Medicine*, 51 (1306): 23–33. https://www.jstor.org/stable/1645011

Wold, B. & Mittelmark, M. B. 2018. Health-promotion research over three decades: The social-ecological model and challenges in implementation of interventions. *Scandinavian Journal of Public Health*, 46 (20): 20–26. https://doi.org/10.1177/1403494817743893

World Health Organization. 1978. *Declaration of Alma Ata*. Geneva: World Health Organization. https://www.who.int/teams/social-determinants-of-health/declaration-of-alma-ata
World Health Organization. 1986. *Ottawa Charter for Health Promotion*. Geneva: World Health Organization. http://www.who.int/healthpromotion/conferences/previous/ottawa/en/
World Health Organization. 1991. *Sundsvall Statement on Supportive Environments for Health*. Geneva: World Health Organization. https://www.who.int/publications/i/item/WHO-HED-92.1
World Health Organization. 1997. *The Jakarta Declaration*. Geneva: World Health Organization. https://www.who.int/publications/i/item/WHO-HPR-HEP-4ICHP-BR-97.4
World Health Organization. 2013. *The Helsinki Statement on Health in All Policies*. The 8th Global Conference on Health Promotion; June 10–14, 2013. https://www.who.int/publications/i/item/9789241506908
World Health Organization. 2017. Promoting health in the SDGs. Report on the 9th Global Conference on Health Promotion, Shanghai, China, 21–24 November 2016: All for health, Health for all. Geneva: World Health Organization.

2

PLANNING TRADITIONS AND PUBLIC HEALTH POLICIES

This chapter uses the instrumental versus communicative dichotomy, and the actor versus structure dichotomy, to classify different political governing systems and to clarify their perspectives on planning, participation, partnerships, policymaking, legitimacy and capacity. The chapter shows that the perspectives have undergone a cumulative process where new perspectives have not replaced but supplemented the old ones. The purpose of this chapter is to clarify the conditions for implementing HiAP as a collaborative legitimizing and capacity building process under different governing systems.

Introduction

Governing systems shape the actors and influence what becomes appropriate processes, actors and actions. At the same time, the actors influence the structures through attitudes and actions and thus create different forms of governing. Therefore, we discuss how different coordination systems as institutional structural forces, or paradigms as Torfing, Sørensen and Røiseland (2016) call them, form the conditions for how public planning, participation, partnership, policymaking and how HiAP can be practiced. We start with presenting the cumulative thoughts and perspective on organizations and public administration which also is found in the theory on governing systems and planning.

William Richard Scott (2002) sees the rise of organization theory in a historical perspective. He finds four dominant theoretical models with representative theories when he combined the dichotomies: closed and open systems and rational and natural systems. Historically the perspectives have moved from seeing organizations as (1) closed and rational systems (1900–1930), (2) closed and

DOI: 10.4324/9781003451273-2

natural (1930–1960), (3) open and rational (1960–1970) and (4) open and natural (1970–present). Many other researchers have made similar classifications as Scott (2002). With special relevance to this chapter, Bukve (1997) uses Scott's four types of organizations on public administration and call the types for (1) rational machine, (2) grown organisms, (3) adapted system and (4) multi-actor systems. Bukve (1997) concludes that in practice they are all in use today, but they are suited for different situations. Compared to Scott (2002), Bukve uses the terms machine and organism instead of rational and natural. We regard this as a distinction between instrumental and communicative rationality. Bukve maintains Scott's distinction between open and closed systems, which we regard as a distinction between actor and structure. See Table 2.1.

A general objection can be raised against using organizational theory, which has largely been developed for private companies, as a perspective on public administration (Christensen et al., 2002). Private companies normally have financial surplus and survival on the market as overriding goals. Public administration is anchored in democratic processes and normally has far more complex objectives and functions in an area of society where, as a rule, no real market exists, but with a need for government and public services. However, reforms in public sector have narrowed the difference between private and public sector, and the reforms in the public sector have not, in our opinion, made this use of organization theory less professionally sound, and we show that the trends that have characterize

TABLE 2.1 Four perspectives on planning in public domain and governing systems

	Closed system perspective *Conservative political ideology* *Endogen factors and power, actors and voluntarism*	*Open system perspective* *Radical political ideology* *Exogen factors and power, structures and determinism*
Rational systems **Instrumental rationality** **Societal guidance** **Process and results are predictable**	Organizations and government as rational machines Policy Analyses tradition Traditional Public Administration	Organizations and government as adaptive systems Social Reform tradition New Public Management
Natural systems **Communicative rationality** **Societal transformation** **Process and results are unpredictable**	Organizations and government as grown organisms Social Learning tradition New Public Governance – conservative	Organizations and government as multi-actor systems Social Mobilization tradition New Public Governance – radical

Source: Based on Friedmann (1987), Scott (2002), Bukve (1997) and Bryson, Crosby and Bloomberg (2014).

organization theory and public administration, are important in planning theory and the distinction between planning traditions.

Classifying theoretical traditions in planning based on the two dichotomies

The instrumental versus communicative rationality dichotomy

Alexander claims that rationality is a prerequisite for all planning and means by that: "Rational planning is planning that has and can give reasons justifying a course of action" (Alexander, 2000: 243). However, rationality is not only an issue in planning. Rationality generally applies to the actors' relationships to the world and how a person perceives and behaves towards his surroundings. Rationality is being able to act in a way that stands up to criticism. A minimum norm for rationality is that there is a match between what the person intends and what the person does. Rationality implies a reflexive attitude, an ability to fulfil knowledge requirements, to learn and to correct behaviour.

The instrumental rationality is the logic of *the traditional linear model of planning*. In this model, the focus is on relating means (how to do thing) to ends (what could be achieved), in logical and systematic ways. Scientific knowledge shall provide an objective basis for identifying present problems and predicting future possibilities (see Figure 2.1). A prerequisite for this planning is, among other things, that when making decisions there is full awareness of the present situation and clear and unambiguous objectives for the future, so that it is possible to choose which alternative offers the best course of action (Simon, 1957).

The instrumental rationality is strongly connected with the *positivists' theory of knowledge*. The presumption here is that objective knowledge can be gained through a scientific, hypothetical-deductive process. The controlled experiment

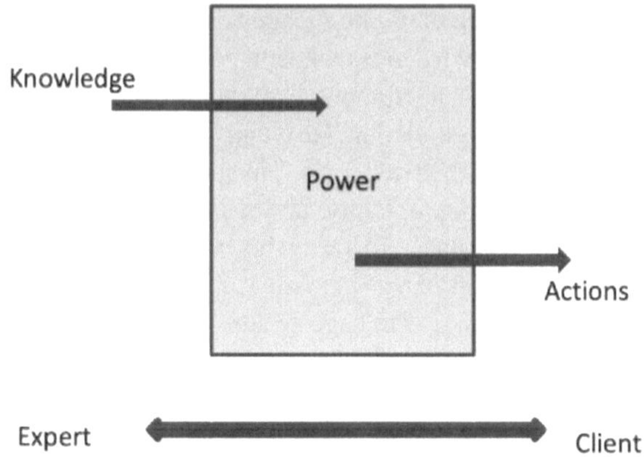

FIGURE 2.1 The positivist epistemology and instrumental planning

Source: Amdam (2010: 20).

stands as the methodical ideal. The origin doctrine for positivism is to clear the world of religion and mysticism, and to achieve control of the society through knowledge and technique. The only true views of the world are those, which are based on empirical observations. Assertions, which are not testable in an analytical or empirical way, shall be disregarded entirely. This positivist science ideal causes an interest towards research aimed at unveiling connections between cause and effect and establishing power based on causality and evidence. Such knowledge can be used to determine the action needed. The instrumental rationality has a strong position in the public health, and is decisive when the society need evidence-based knowledge to intervene in processes in order to prevent people from illness and injuries.

Friedmann (1978) states that the positivist epistemology is based on the definition of objective knowledge that is independent of any knowing subject, and that the epistemology is too dominating in our time. Schön (1986) argues likewise and claims that this epistemology has led to practise as an instrumental professional activity where the process of solving problems is made rigorous using science, theory and technique. The owners of the scientific knowledge have formed professions based on the following characteristics: basic knowledge, used science and action competence. Some of these actors have through use of the positivist science ideal made systemized bases of knowledge with four important capabilities. The knowledge is *specialized, stabilized, standardized* and *scientific*. These actors have made what Schön calls *over-professions* based on instrumental rationality and codified knowledge (medical doctors, engineers, etc.). Some of the other actors can be called *under-professions*. We say that typical examples of these under-professions can be planners, public health and social workers and any other who base their knowledge on participation in social interaction. These professions are not capable of making a basis for systematic scientific knowledge, because the same actions will give different results in different contexts. Their competence of action is weak because the coherence between their knowledge and actions is complex and labile, and much of the adequate knowledge is tacit, and personally and locally embedded.

Schön (1983) suggests that instrumental rationality is a process for problem-solving, but not for problem-formulating. He claims this by saying that instrumental models of action do not catch the real world. The model cannot handle uncertainty in forms of non-stability and complexity, and it is not capable of handling conflicting needs, interests and values. Towards the end, Schön ads that instrumental rationality is not the only point of view existing, there are other competing forms of rationality. Schön (1983) asks us to eagerly admit the weaknesses of instrumental rationality and rather seek for an epistemology which is based upon practice in creativity and intuitiveness similar to that what the practitioners use when they face unique situations with uncertainty, conflicts and instability. Schön introduces and uses the word *reflective practitioner*, and writes that when one reflects during actions, one becomes researcher in a practical context. One does not depend upon theories or techniques; one makes theory out of cases. This rationality is suitable for handling uncertainty because it does not separate ends and means, knowledge and actions, planning and implementation from each other. They are all developed interactively. After a while one will have both a *codified* and a *tacit knowledge* that one base one's actions upon. However, the tacit knowledge can be a weakness with the reflective practitioners. Specialists, for instance, have a great deal of uncodified tacit knowledge based on earlier experiences. Thus, they can be regarded as boring, exhausted and over-educated, and they can also become dragged into patterns of action with mistakes they cannot correct, and therefore become inattentive to situations not fitting into their established patterns of actions. The reflective practitioner must therefore involve him- or herself with communicative situations where these irrational actions can be revealed and corrected.

Schön (1986) does not refer to Friedmann's work, but the intention of Friedmann (1978) was also to make an alternative epistemology for use in social contexts as a substitute for the epistemology occupied with objective knowledge based on the positivist science ideal. Friedmann (1978) discards the positivist science ideal, and thus also the deductive research design's approach to obtain objective knowledge through verifying and falsifying of hypotheses. Friedmann put forward the *epistemology of social practice* as an alternative to the positivist epistemology. Friedmann writes that this epistemology can be traced back to Aristotle because social practice refers to moral actions in public spheres, and because actions are based on norms regarding how one is supposed to live along with each other. In this model, learning is linked to events via social actions and the results of that action. The adequacy of the theory of reality is therefore dependent on the results of action and the extent to which these results satisfy the given social values. The social practice epistemology is a model for *social learning* where the learning happens with interaction between changed practice and new recognition (see model in Figure 2.2).

In this model, knowledge and action can be linked through critical understanding and radical practice, and the planning process is a far-reaching learning process in which everyone can participate. Friedmann argues for a constant critical evaluation and successive revision of the components in the model, and maintains that without a vision there is no radical practice, without radical practice no formation

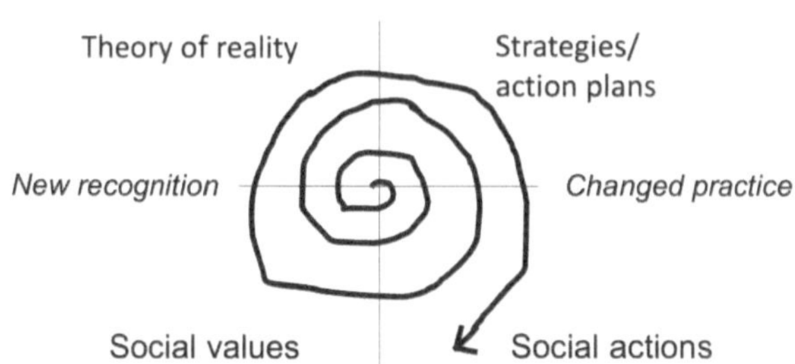

FIGURE 2.2 The social practice epistemology and communicative planning

Source: Based on Friedmann (1978: 87) and Amdam (2010: 23).

of a theory, without a theory no strategy and without a strategy no action. Friedmann points out the following advantages of this model (1978: 87):

- Knowledge and actions can be tied to a model for democratic processes.
- Knowledge grows from conflicting incidents and thus has a political dimension.
- Anyone who wants to can participate, and there exists no monopoly or distinguished elite.
- The separation between objective and subjective knowledge disappears, and abstract and concrete knowledge is combined in a single process of learning and practising.
- Normative contributions will not be smuggled in but will openly be presented for criticism.
- The model can be used in formulations of theories. What is learned in one situation can be abstract knowledge in another.

The model shows that social practice grows through a continuous critical evaluation and successive revision of the components in the model as they malfunction. The model results in *personal growth* because the participants tie together knowledge and actions when they alter between critical acknowledging and new practice in the collaborative process. However, Friedmann admits that even if the epistemology regarding social practice exceeds the epistemology dealing with objective knowledge, it is far from a substituted.

Friedmann gets support for his ideas about the social practice epistemology by among others Bolan (1980) who writes about the *practitioner as theorist*. He also starts by saying that the difference between theory and practice, knowledge and actions is bigger than ever. He asserts further that if one makes planning a professional and instrumental problem-solver, one effect could be that citizens would become less self-sufficient and that they would come into a structural relationship of dependency towards professional helpers. This effect could eventually become stronger, making the distance between knowledge and actions even greater. He maintains that every incident is special, and the most meaningful theories are those that are constructed in the minds of the practitioners and that have been tried out in practice. He says that professional practice is guided by knowledge and that knowledge is formed by practice. However, norms, interests and values control actions, thus, the planner should not only be regarded as an instrumental planner, but also as a communicative politician representing norms, interests and values.

Communicative planning is rooted in the epistemology of social practice and is not carried out by experts for the object of the plan, but in face-to-face dialogue between those involved and interested (Healey, 1997, 2003). Communicative planning has a pragmatic perspective on the dichotomy and maintains that in practice instrumental and communicative rationality is combined. Personal growth and joint action are the key elements in communicative planning. Rather than a technocratic process carried out by planners, planning is regarded as an interactive communicative process (Innes & Booher, 2004), and the planning process shall transform knowledge into action through an uninterrupted sequence of relationships between people (Friedmann, 1992). The planning shall not be divorced from other social action in which the aim is to gain control over social processes that effect one's welfare. Communicative planning emphasizes a broad grass-root mobilization to gain the strength to take greater responsibility for one's development and to influence the conditions under which one is working, and it is assumed that better decisions are reached if they emerge out of a dialogue between those concerned.

The actor versus structure dichotomy

Actor versus structure is often portrayed as a real dichotomy, but what is discussed most are the relationships between them. One can understand actors' actions as individual exercise of power, but the distribution of power between individuals in society is governed by social structures. Therefore, the term actor versus structure has many parallels in pairs of terms such as individual and society, voluntarism and determinism, endogenous and exogenous explained development and considering organizations and institutions as closed systems with weak exogenous influence and open systems with strong exogenous influence. In public health, this dichotomy is best known through the work of Dahlgren and Whitehead (1991) and their *model for social determinants of health*. The model places people's actions and characteristics such as age, gender and constitutional factors in the centre, and individual living habits, social networks and social support, living and working conditions and general socio-economic conditions as influencing factors around the centre. The model tells us that a person's actions are affected by the determinants, but that the choices one makes in sum can strengthen or weaken the determinants.

Giddens (1984) has with his works on *structuration theory* contributed a lot to clarifying the relationships between actors and structures. The aim of his structuration theory is to abolish the dichotomy between objectivist and subjectivist understanding of social practice, and to explain how societies are organized and integrated in time and space. His main message is that actors and structures mutually influence each other. He writes that the structuration is within us. We confirm, challenge, or change the moral-forming structural forces, and through that process we change ourselves and our culture. This means in plain text that when we can create structures, we can also change them if we want. To build such moral-forming collectives demands that the people participate as "whole" people who are concerned with the common good, and not as calculating experts advancing their own interests. Therefore, strong and active civil societies and social networks are decisive arenas for building the moral collectives; see among others Putnam (1993). Moral collectives help to create the trust between people that is necessary to encourage them to take a stand for the collective without fear of being exploited by persons who are simply out to promote their own interests, without considering the consequences for the collectives they are a part of.

In the planning theory Friedmann (1992) joins the criticism of the modernization of society and argues that a relative strengthening of the instrumental rationality is taking place in private enterprises and public sector administration. He believes that this has a negative effect on the communicative common sense, which in the main is kept alive in the democratic elected governing bodies and in the civil society. Developing this argument further, he claims that the modernization has led to an increased emphasis on instrumental rationality and the promoting of self-interest, with less emphasis being placed on a fellowship that forms morals and on collective interests. Friedmann believes the key to further development now is to strengthen the relations between the social power in the civil society and the political power in the democratically elected governing bodies. Furthermore, he maintains that politics should lead to the formation of a moral fellowship and that political activity therefore cannot be reduced to the economic calculation of the utilitarian value and sociological determinism. In this way strengthening of the *horizontal power structure* through activating the civil society, the elected representatives and private businesses in collaborative processes, the horizontal political power can be organized to supplement and oppose the sector dominated and *vertical power structure.*

But Friedmann himself is aware that the strengthening of relations between the civil society and the people's democratically elected representatives often meets strong opposition from the established government power, and a two-parallel planning system seems to become both logical and desirable (Friedmann, 1992; Zoete, 2000; Amdam, 2002). It becomes logical that the territorial planning which in general emphasizes cross-sectoral spatial development, in the main is carried out in informal network organizations based on the public, private and voluntary sectors. Moreover, that the sector-based public planning, which in general is a planning of sector activities, is carried out within the domains of the formal government organizations, but that this planning both receives and delivers premises for the territorial planning. Or to put it another way, the challenge of the territorial public planning is to get organizations in the public, private and voluntary sectors to participate in the network organizations or partnerships that the territorial local and regional planning manages to establish. Thus, territorial planning needs to become an institutional capacity building process (Healey, 1997; Healey, de Magalhaes & Mandipour, 1999). The local and regional planning and development organizations must be regarded as legitimate and must be accepted by the public, private and voluntary sectors and by local, regional and national levels of government. In contrast to the sector organizations, these territorial partnership organizations cannot be given legitimacy from a superior institution in the political power structure, because no one seem to have the full and necessary cross-sector legitimacy in relation to the regional and local planning and development work. Local and regional political partnerships must therefore create their legitimacy and political power through planning processes.

Four planning traditions in the public domain based on the two dichotomies

In 1987, John Friedmann published a book in which he in an exemplary manner, compiles various contributions to the development of planning in the public domain. Thoughts and perspectives on organization is a major contributor to the classification of the traditions, which are *Policy Analysis*, *Social Reform*, *Social Learning* and *Social Mobilization* (see Table 2.1). We regard his classification of planning traditions in the public domain as fundamental, and it provides a broad theoretical discussion of what planning is and should be.

Friedmann (1987: 36) claims that in planning one is faced with a meta-theoretical problem: how to effectively get technical/professional knowledge to be the basis for people's choice of actions. In the discussion of the problem, he firstly distinguishes between public planning as *social guidance* and as *social transformation* in the view of how knowledge is linked to action:

- In public *planning as social guidance* the emphasis is placed on ideals such as objective knowledge and causality between activities and effects. Therefore, one perceives connections between knowledge and action as an instrumental, and presupposes fine-tuned harmony between actors so that the planning subject has sufficient control to implement its decisions. This form of planning has dominated much of public planning.
- This form stands in contrast to *planning as social transformation* where knowledge is seen as an integrated part of action. Emphasis is placed on communication and learning through practice, and that behaviour can be changed, and that theories are made valid in practice. This form of planning is often actualized in crisis situations, when the legitimate authority of the state is weak, and when the state does not hold strong political power.

Secondly, he divides between extremes in the view of the state as the ruler of society. With threads back to the Vienna circle, with Comte and especially Bentham, Friedmann (1987) believes he can identify a conservative/liberal and a radical ideological direction in how knowledge can be linked to action.

- In *conservative and liberal political ideology*, there is a record of how public planning can serve the power apparatus in society, which should ideally build its power on free actors who, through their rational choices, can express their wishes through markets and democracy. In politics, he recognizes this as an ideological foundation for the right-wing side, which believes that actors' free choice of actions and the least possible government interference can lead to the good society.

- This contrasts with *the radical political ideology*, which is more concerned with the structural constraints on the exercise of free choice, and with changes in power relations in society. Here lies the foundation for the political left, which believes that to realize the good society for all, power structures must be changed so that all actors have equal opportunities to make free choices of actions.

We interpret Friedmann (1987) so that one can achieve social guidance through instrumental rationality when the goals are clear and accepted, when one has the knowledge to calculate our way to the best actions, and when one has the power to control the implementation (rational systems). Furthermore, that social transformation through communicative rationality is only fully developed in dialogues (natural systems). In addition, we interpret Friedmann (1987) so that the distinction between the conservative and radical ideology reflects whether the planning is exercised in a situation where the planning unit has great freedom of choice to promote voluntary behaviour (closed system view), or in a situation where the environment largely limits the actors' possibilities for action (open system view). Consequently, we add these characteristics to Friedmann's four traditions:

1 The Policy Analysis tradition (instrumental rationality and closed system view)
2 The Social Reform tradition (instrumental rationality and open system view)
3 The Social Learning tradition (communicative rationality and closed system view)
4 The Social Mobilization tradition (communicative rationality and open system view)

Based on the discussion so far, we can distinguish between situations suitable for instrumental rationality (having solid causal knowledge that makes process and result predictable) and communicative rationality (lacking causal knowledge that makes process and result unpredictable). Furthermore, we can distinguish between situations where endogenous forces are decisive for development (great power over one's own situation), and where exogenous forces are decisive for development (little power over one's own situation). Then we get four situations with relation to the planning traditions. See Table 2.1.

Four planning traditions and governing systems

In the governing of the society, using the state, the market and networks as coordination systems have been emphasized differently over time (Bryson, Crosby & Bloomberg, 2014). These coordination systems have formed institutional structures in the form of a hierarchical public administration system that promotes efficiency, a market-based management system that will also promote effectiveness, and a network-based governance system where stakeholders are mutual dependent in delivering efficiency, effectiveness and quality. These institutional structures are named competing paradigms for public governance and leadership (Hartley, 2005; Bouckaert, Peters & Verhoest, 2010: 28 and 29). Bryson, Crosby and Bloomberg (2014) similarly identify characteristics of three different approaches to public administration:

- *Traditional Public Administration* (TPA) organized as a Weberian bureaucracy with a hierarchical and commanding leadership function and a distinction between expert and client. TPA is based on rule-management, hierarchy and professional judgement. This governing system bases its legitimacy on input and output (laws and regulations, research-based knowledge, resource distribution, completed activities, etc.).
- *New Public Management* (NPM) is based on an ordering-and-executioner model, a result-oriented management function and a distinction between provider and customer. NPM places emphasis on target and results management, customers and market thinking and on outcome legitimacy in the form of concrete objectives achieved. Nevertheless, the public sector under this governing system has become more divided, and the units have been focused on achieving their production targets, rather than on effects and consequences for individuals and across the units. The results are increased unit-egoism, silo-thinking and fragmentation.
- The emergence of *New Public Governance* (NPG) can be seen as a response to NPM (Osborne, 2009). In this governing system actors are organized in networks of mutually dependent and equal actors. Here, citizen participation is emphasized, and one important leadership function is to create good inclusive and reflective processes. Here, fragmentation, silo-thinking and the selfish actions of the various units are seen as part of the problem, and the solution is a collaboration between multi-actors in networks with an emphasis on processes and achieving outcome legitimacy. A legitimacy that is achieved through satisfying needs and creating public values. Democracy, citizenship and skilled citizens who engage in conscious problem-solving are central public values in this governing system.

In our interpretation the TPA belongs to the Analyses Tradition, and the NPM belongs to the Reform Tradition. Further, the NPG is overlapping with Friedmann's Social Transformation perspective with the Social Learning and Social Mobilizing traditions which are instituted on and separated by the conservative and the radical ideology. See Tables 2.1 and 2.2. Based on this, we argue that NPG can be divided into two variants. A conservative variant where the focus is on the communicative processes between independent actors who across governing levels and sectors are part of voluntary collaborations, and a radical variant which utilizes the opportunities to influence and change the structures that counteract collaborations and the satisfaction of needs. The conservative variant is based on the learning tradition and means that relevant actors come together voluntarily to co-produce services

TABLE 2.2 Governing system and public health politics

Traditional Public Administration (TPA)	*New Public Management (NPM)*	*New Public Governance (NPG) – conservative*	*New Public Governance (NPG) – radical*
Key elements:	*Key elements:*	*Key elements:*	*Key elements:*
Instrumental rationality and closed systems Hierarchy and government	Instrumental rationality and open systems Market and government	Communicative rationality and closed systems Network and governance	Communicative rationality and open systems Network and governance
Political theory and naïve social sciences Rule management and authority Instrumental linear planning	Economic theory of self-utilization Goal management, contracting and control Incremental planning	Democratic theory and learning theory Value-based management Negotiating planning	Democratic theory and empowerment Value-conscious management Transactive planning
Expert / service providers manage clients Participation is open to all, but priority to the affected	Customers influence service providers Participation from customers and user representatives	Service providers and citizens as co-producers Participation from active users	Service providers and citizens as co-creators Participation from political active citizens
Input legitimacy Efficiency (equal treatment of clients)	Output legitimacy Efficiency and effectiveness (satisfied customers)	Outcome legitimacy Efficiency, effectiveness and quality (supporting the needs)	Impact legitimacy Efficiency, effectiveness, quality and legitimacy (fulfil purpose/societal values)
Capacity for direct societal intervention based on laws, regulations and evidence-based knowledge Changes are dependent on a change in political leadership	Capacity for indirect societal steering based on goals and results Changes are dependent on new political goals and values	Capacity for community development based on partnerships within established power structures Changes depend on the actors in the partnerships' competence and willingness to cooperate	Capacity for societal development based on partnerships that challenge established power structures Changes are dependent on structural framework conditions and the partners' capacity to change them
Public health policy: Demanding use of security equipment, forbidding unhealthy activities, etc.	**Public health policy:** Stimulating healthy activities. Make unhealthy activities less affordable	**Public health policy:** Teaching/learning people to make healthy choices and to change their way of living	**Public health policy:** Mobilize people to change their way of living and their living conditions (the health determinants)

Source: Based on Friedmann (1987) and Bryson, Crosby and Bloomberg (2014).

within the framework that applies to each actor. They represent the established power structure. This variant may be sufficient to deliver increased efficiency, effectiveness and quality, but co-production will never be more than a common minimum of what the various actors can contribute within the interpretation of applicable laws, regulations and objectives. This in contrast to the radical variant which intends to change the structural conditions through local mobilization and bottom-up politics. For this governing system, the basic understanding is that actors and structures mutually influence each other, and that when humans have created the structures, they can also change them.

The Policy Analysis tradition and Traditional Public Administration

Friedmann (1987) characterizes the Policy Analysis tradition by more faith in objective science, even if it is not perfect, than in politics with emotions and irrationality. The elected representatives represent the people and are sovereign, and the administration must be a neutral instrument for the elected representatives. Political theories predominate, and what are the interests of the people are determined by elected officials and professional experts. The society is governed by command based on laws, regulations and decisions. Further characteristics are the belief in the planners as neutral technocrats, and in perfect markets and democracy.

In the Policy Analysis tradition instrumental rationality and closed system view with focus on endogen factors dominate. In this tradition, organizations and administrations are regarded as rational machines. This perspective represents early organizational theory and perceives all organizations as similar and understands management as the practice of special functions and roles. This means that organizations are classified as formal and closed, and they are perceived as social units that are deliberately constructed and reconstructed to realize specific goals. For the administration, this means that the employees are organized, specialized and socialized to perform established functions, implement the decisions, and promote the wishes of those in power. Changes express the opinions of those in power. Organizational behaviour is goal-oriented and autonomous, and the managers try to be proactive.

The perception is that the best solution can be calculated, and planning can be instrumental and linear within a closed system. The synoptic or *rational planning* belongs to this tradition. This form of planning is often presented as an ideal model for planning, but the model is also an ideal on which many other academic traditions are based, among others in economics and organizational theory (Simon, 1957). Within planning, it is Banfield (1973) who has most clearly formulated the requirements for such planning, which is also called normative, analytical and synoptic. The planning process is seen as a step-by-step and linear work where one sequentially:

1 Formulates clear and unambiguous goals
2 Formulates and analyses all possible action alternatives

3 Prepares all possible actions of all alternatives
4 Considers the consequences
5 Determines which alternative has effects (consequences) that best meet the previously determined goals
6 Implements the selected option
7 Compiles experience and results for use in new decision-making situations

From practical planning we know that these ideal conditions can never be fully present (Simon, 1957). In addition, the planning process is here based on a clear division of roles between planners and politicians. The politicians are responsible for phase 1 and 5. Planning according to this tradition is limited to phases 2, 3 and 4. The implementation of the chosen alternative and learning is usually not seen as a planning task. This tradition emphasizes decision-making and not implementation, and this separation is put forward as a serious criticism of this form of planning (Friedmann, 1987).

The most extreme form of instrumental planning does not have room for participation because professional experts are supposed to have the knowledge and power to formulate both the understanding and the solving of problems. As far as participation is concerned, it is presented as a ladder with low degree of participation at the bottom and high degree of participation at the top (Arnstein, 1969). In principle, everyone can participate, but it is still up to the public governing bodies to decide how much the actors can influence the results. However, there is often a conflict between the experts' professional knowledge and the lay people's local knowledge, and most commonly the experts and elected officials decide how much weight the local knowledge should be added.

This tradition dominates what is called TPA which is based on Weberian bureaucracy with hierarchical and commanding rule management with a distinction between expert and client, and entities in this bureaucracy has clearly delineated responsibilities (Hartley, 2005). According to Bryson, Crosby and Bloomberg (2014: 226), the basic understanding of TPA is an ideal instrumental rationality with a utility-maximizing human being. TPA gives the public sector power to control developments in the private and voluntary sectors. The governing system runs as bureaucracy with an orderly hierarchy and a central power to control and command but is criticized for creating clients and being bureaucratic in a negative sense (Allmendinger, 2009). The accountability is hierarchical so that employees are responsible upward in the hierarchy and ultimately for the elected officials. These elected officials are the most important actors in the political processes, and they define what is public interest and common good. The actual decisions are taken by elected officials in the representative democracy, and the citizens have a right to participate indirectly through electoral schemes or directly through participation. The elected officials are responsible to the citizens who can replace them at the next election. The inhabitants are regarded as voters, constituents and clients. In TPA the governing system has the power to design and implement policies limiting people's choice of actions, and the democratic legitimacy is based on political decided laws and regulations, resource allocations, etc. The main source of this formal input legitimacy is the representative democracy and the parliamentary chain of governance. This governing system emphasizes high *efficiency* meaning to produce in the right way with optimal utilization of resources and equal treatment of clients (see Chapter 1).

Summing up the tradition and presenting its public health politics

In summary, the Policy Analysis tradition and TPA is mainly based on an instrumental rationality and perceives the public administration as a coordinated actor with great opportunities to manage society as the elected politicians want. Public sector has the power to manage development in the private and voluntary sector and to intervene directly in people's everyday life (the intervening state). Practising TPA draws planning in the direction of synoptic and linear forms of planning with a sharp distinction between elected officials and administrative staff, and where elected officials formulate goals and regulations, and where the administration examines the situation, solutions and consequences. The scope of planning in this governing system is the administration of law, with emphasis on taking care of all the inhabitants' interests in the best possible way. The planning and participation process is expert-driven form of planning that aims to gather knowledge so that elected officials can adopt the best possible plans that coordinate resources and care for those involved. The participants' degree of impact on the plan depends on the contributors' position of power and how the professional and political leaders consider their contributions.

Accountability in this planning tradition and governing system emphasizes whether the different public sector units produce in the right way and can make HiAP able to contribute to increased production and efficiency (outputs). Example of such public health policy is demands supported with laws and regulations about using security equipment in cars, at work etc., forbidding unhealthy activities such as smoking, and restricting the use of pesticides and additives in the foods production. However, these interventions must be legitimate and there must be causality between the activity and the effects, which can be transformed to evidence-based political intervening practice. However, the process to reach these legitimated interventions in people's activities can be a long and complicated discussion about facts and causalities, prioritizing interests, and what matters for people and their health. Thus, this tradition and governing system will not be able to handle public health as a wicked problem.

The Social Reform tradition and New Public Management

The Social Analysis tradition and the Social Reform tradition are both instrumental, but the second tradition emphasizes more the uncertainty that comes from changes over time and the forces in society than the first. Organizations are regarded as adapted systems and organizational behaviour is deterministic, forced and adaptive, and the leaders often become reactive. The Social Reform Tradition practices top-down political management in the form of stimulation or obstructing ongoing development processes in society based on accepted overarching goals. According to this tradition, it becomes important for policymaking to influence the actors so that they act in line with what the policymakers expect and demand.

In the Social Reform tradition instrumental rationality and open system view with focus on exogen factors dominate and draws public planning towards experimental and *incremental planning* where one tries to find solutions, but which constantly must be corrected. This incremental small-step planning is experimental in that it tries out different tools to reach the target, and then it uses the means with best effects. Lindblom (1959) presents his model "muddling through" as disjointed incrementalism, and as a planning theory which he believes is closer to the political reality than the rational model. This planning implies a process where one makes small steps forward, corrects both goals and means, and continuously tries to work one's way forward towards overall values. Lindblom (1959) emphasizes that such fundamental values and goals always exist in a society, such as full employment and economic growth, even if they are not always clearly stated in politics.

Public participation in the incremental planning is practiced mainly through user surveys, participation in user boards at schools and kindergartens and user representatives in governing bodies at hospitals and other institutions. Furthermore, if a single service recipient has the capacity to contribute, he or she can influence the service providers. Furthermore, action groups may arise and argue based on alternative understandings of the situation. For public planning, it is therefore important to obtain knowledge about such user experiences and alternative understandings, and to take account of them in the planning. It is especially important if users' demands and expectations for the public sector are unrealistically high.

The modernization of the public sector since 1980 have had this tradition as a reform ideal, and the tradition is expressed through NPM. This governing system emerged as a reaction to the TPA, which was criticized for being too bureaucratic, regulated, slow and inefficient. Bryson, Crosby and Bloomberg (2014: 446) write that NPM assumes that human beings are instrumentally rational (Simon, 1957), and that the governing system is dominated by economics theories in which the interests of the people are determined by the elected officials, or by aggregating people's individual preferences. Further, the system is based on ordering and execution models, goals and results management, and a distinction between provider and customer. The elected officials are important in policymaking but appointed administrative leaders have been delegated political power.

Public sector is regarded as a marked where the state must promote the overall goals in the society by means of indirect governing (the regulating state). The administration must appear as an adapted system where roles and positions are placed in a hierarchy with the aim of being an efficient system, and changes take place as an adaptation to the environment. This means that the politicians can promote desirable actions and inhibiting undesirable actions using reforms, regulations and goal and result management. Hence, national initiated reforms are commonly used to achieve changes in school, health and other public sectors.

With its market-oriented assumptions, this tradition is expected to be particularly suitable for public service production. Thus, the residents must be given the opportunity to choose between private and public providers, and between different public providers. The citizens are considered customers, and even if they do not pay with their own money, the public funds follow with the choices they make. However, such quasi-markets easily lead to what is called target displacement, in that production is aligned with the targets to be reported on, in the hope that this will legitimize the use of resources.

NPM reforms have been a significant driving force in the transformation of public sector. The label New Public Management was first used by Hood (1991) to describe a public sector modernization reform wave which spreads rapidly to many countries. The main hypothesis in the reforms is that more market, more management and greater autonomy will produce more efficiency without having negative side-effects on other public sector values. However, the promised impacts and effects are seldom much documented (Pollitt, 2002).

In NPM one tries to give managers and their subordinates more autonomy and to strengthen political control through contracts, monitoring and incentive systems at the same time. But, reduced political control is the most significant consequence from the NPM reform (Pollitt & Bouckaert, 2000; Christensen & Lægreid, 2004). There seem to be an anti-political trend that potentially can undermine political control, because the devolution has increased the distance between the political leadership and the subordinate units and lower levels of management. There is a tendency to define political involvement in public enterprises as "inappropriate" interference in business matters (Christensen & Lægreid, 2004).

The introduction of management by objectives and results approach from private sector into public sector is a central element in NPM. Those who have evaluated this management tool do not hesitate to characterize it as a large and complicated, control-oriented system (Christensen et al., 2002: 100). Their research underpins the fact that the reform has been characterized by relatively highly detailed requirements for describing goals, performance indicators and measures and requiring formalized, written reporting between administrative units and levels. The result has been a compromise between classic bureaucratic government and modern forms of goal management. Christensen et al. (2002) further report that management by objectives and results functions better as administrative control over subordinate bodies than as capability for political governance.

Through the NPM reform wave, the public administration is simultaneously trying to achieve both greater control and more freedom, but these intentions are difficult to achieve simultaneously (Pollitt & Bouckaert, 2000), leading to significant consequences such as increased vertical and horizontal specialization and fragmentation. Authority is transferred downwards in the hierarchy, either between existing organizations or to new governmental organizations, both inside and outside the governmental administrative organization. The idea is to separate politics from administrational and service producing functions, and to make public sector more like private sector. This vertical specialization has often gone hand in hand with the horizontal specialization. Here, functions that were traditionally organized together and with direct political control, such as policy advice, regulative tasks, ownership functions, control functions and purchaser/provider functions, have now been separated into distinct units and often on an "arm's length" from the politicians.

The NPM reforms intended to empower customers through free chooses of services, to free managers from detailed political instructions, and to strengthen political steering through defining the long-term goals for the public sector and asserting the outcome. The public sector is given a hybrid character that draws both towards centralization and decentralization, which leads to fragmentation of power and responsibility, and thus little holistic thinking, poor satisfaction of needs and poor quality of services. The consequence is a fragmentation of the national stats and an increased sector thinking and acting (Christensen & Lægreid, 2004: 13).

NPM wants to promote both *efficiency* and *effectiveness* (see Chapter 1), but research indicates that this governance system has neither resulted in better efficiency nor effectiveness (Hood & Dixon, 2015). NPM is fundamentally instrumental in its logic, and thus presupposes an instrumental rationality with causal connections between cause and effect, and thus between effort (input), activities (output) and results in the form of effects and qualities (outcome). In practice, this condition is difficult to fulfil. Firstly, it is more difficult to measure the effects of activities, and secondly, it is more difficult to establish statistical and logical connections between efforts and effects (outcome), than between efforts and activity (output). Consequently, the actors and organizations in the public sector are more engaged in producing outputs in line with financial frameworks, standards, manuals and procedures that are beneficial for their unit, than producing outcomes that are beneficial for the society. The upshot is what one calls *unity egoism*, which weakens *societal responsibility* in the public sector and poses a major challenge, especially for collaborative planning in which public, private and voluntary sectors are expected to cooperate and contribute to the desired societal development.

NPM has therefore resulted in a rigid control system, unit selfishness, a search for standard procedures, mistrust and reduced professional discretion, which means that the satisfaction of needs and the effects of the various units' actions on individuals and society have been largely overlooked. Citizens having enough resources to present their needs is an important *threshold* for public service users in NPM, and if citizens come across this obstacle and stand in *queue*, they often find that when they reach the *counter* it was a wrong queue. They must move to the back of another queue. Furthermore, because it is important for public sector to have a good reputation based on satisfied citizens it is possible for resourceful users to engage both lawyers and media (*voice*) to promote their interests and get their needs satisfied. In addition, resourceful citizens can choose to exit from public sector services and buy private services. Other less resourceful users choose to *loyally* queue up or respond with *passivity*. Therefore, Hirschman (1970) model "exit, voice and loyalty" give a striking characteristic of this governing system.

Summing up the tradition and presenting its public health politics

Following the Social Reform tradition, planning must be instrumental in an open system, but when the external forces are regarded strong, planning becomes incremental, small step planning with continuous logical adjustment to the situation. This tradition is expressed though the NPM governing system which is based on market thinking and exhibits a conflicting character that draws both towards centralization and towards decentralization, which results in a division of power and responsibility. Furthermore, goal and result management lead to unit-egoism and silo-thinking, which means that satisfying customers with complex needs and solving society's complex and wicked problems are easily displaced.

Accountability in this this planning tradition and governing system emphasizes increased effectiveness in addition to efficiency (see Chapter 1). Effectiveness means whether one produces what is considered the right in relation to the current objectives, and for HiAP this implies creating incentive structures that make people act in accordance with the political given goals, and by using different and continues adjusted means. For example, building infrastructure that promotes physical activity, putting taxes on unhealthy food and reducing taxes on healthy foods, and most important, using the tax system to redistribution of money between poor and rich people to resolve the social gradient where unhealth and poverty follows families and local communities for generations. This public health policy is aimed improving the health determinants to stimulate people to take healthy decisions and thus indirectly improve people's actions and health. However, the utilitarian logic of the various actors seems to cause fragmentation and unit-egoism, and a need to strengthen the logic of norms with communicative forms of planning and management is obvious. This planning tradition and the NPM system have so far been unable to handle public health as a wicked problem.

The emergence of New Public Governance

Osborne (2009) writes that the emergence of NPG is a reaction to the weaknesses of NPM. In NPG, complexity and fragmentation with silo-thinking and unit-selfishness are counted as the very problem, and the solution is innovative multi-actor collaboration in networks with emphasis on democratic processes and on satisfying the needs of the society and strengthening the legitimacy and capacity of the governing body. In NPG communicative logic with demands for equal partners, face-to-face dialogue, and open democratic processes are important issues. Democracy and politically active citizens who engage in conscious problem-solving are central characteristics of NPG.

NPG has a special asset when it comes to dealing with complex and conflicting problems that require participation and collaborative efforts by public, private and voluntary actors. This governing system has focus on a high degree of purpose management, outcome legitimacy and quality in form of satisfaction of needs. Communication is the coordination mechanism, and the organizational form is partnership with voluntary agreements between mutually dependent actors. To succeed, such partnerships require that the actors together manage to come up with new problem understandings and new problem-solving. Thus, NPG requires collaborative forms of planning where the purpose of planning and participation is to stimulate learning and capacity building to exploit and possibly change the structural forces in societies. Thus, NPG demands value-based management and practical judgement (wisdom) in a practice of knowing and learning (Davoudi, 2015). This means that the Ladder of Citizen Participation (Arnstein, 1969) must be replaced by the Spiral of citizen participation (see Chapter 1).

Actors in collaborative partnerships gain capacity to act by blending their resources, skills and purpose into a long term-coalition. Partnerships are therefore complex and dissolvable. They are *complex* because they are made up of organizations that are quite different, but which each contributes to the network with their own speciality. They are *dissolvable* in the sense that participating organizations can be replaced and the network itself can be completely disbanded its strength. Network organizations are often regarded as more innovative and able to handle uncertainty than bureaucratic organizations, but this ought to be handled more as a hypothesis than an axiomatic fact. However, network organizations are normally loosely coupled organizations, and therefore obtain the power and legitimacy the different collaborating organizations want to give them, and the power the context can accept (Strand, 2001).

Participating in network organizations may be motivated on self-interest or based on mutual usefulness and common values, and the collaboration is normally formalized through agreements and transaction control mechanisms between the participants. In theory the control mechanism in network organizations can be based on market, bureaucracy or trust (Langfield-Smith & Smith, 2003: 286), but accountability deficit does often become a problem, because partners in network organizations have a significant degree of autonomy and are driven by the self-interest of their members rather than a wider concern with the public interest and particularly with those excluded from the network (Stoker, 1998: 24). To a certain extent, accountability can be regulated through agreements, but often agreed actions can come to a halt because the actors end up in a cross-pressure between accountability towards the network organization and their own organization, which is often governed according to a combination of TPA and NPM. Sørensen and Torfing (2012) and Torfing (2016) argue that in practice all multi-stakeholder cooperation will be an arena where all three governing systems have their actors. Actors structured by TPA will count the hierarchy as innovation driver, those structured by NPM will count competition as innovation driver and those who believe in NPG will count networking and collaboration as the driver of public sector innovation (Hartley, Sørensen & Torfing, 2013).

As an illustration of this, it is often said that cooperation between sector-silos lives in the shadow of the silos (Scharpf, 1999; Héritier & Lehmkuhl, 2008). This means that the capacity for action and democratic legitimacy that network organizations can achieve, depends on what the government bodies can accept in relation to their laws and regulations in TPA, and their target and result requirements in the NPM. It is expected that the elected officials, the public and private sector employees and other citizens together will formulate goals and measures in collaborative learning processes, and for this they will need a large room for discretion from strict regulations and goals. This means that the extent to which network organizations are empowered to successfully complete their tasks depends partly on the legitimacy they receive from their partners, but mostly on how much legitimacy they manage to build up themselves through the collaboration (Christensen, Lægreid & Rykkja, 2016).

NPG is based on value-conscious and purpose management, and the goal is to improve *efficiency*, *effectiveness* and *quality* through resource mobilization and innovation (Sørensen & Torfing, 2014: 9). We add the goal to *legitimize* the partnership through fulfilment of the partnership's overall purpose with such values as sustainability, social inequality, democracy, etc. (see Chapter 1). Thus, the legitimacy of network organizations dependents on the efficiency, effectiveness and quality they can demonstrate, and to what degree the actual process justifies their existence. Hence, the legitimacy of such an organization will come both from inside and outside. The legitimacy from within will depend on how much power the participating organizations are willing to transfer to the network, and this transfer is normally limited by what is in the interests of the participant at any time. In understanding the acceptance and legitimacy from outside, it is important to stress the fact that network organizations will be involved in a continual competition with other organizations, and that they will challenge the power in the vertical and horizontal power structures in the society. It is therefore vital for the legitimacy of network organizations that the participating organizations act in the networks with powers of attorney that are well supported in their organizations.

Collaboration can be regarded as a prerequisite for NPG, and collaboration in NPG presumes that involved citizens and experts act in networks with the understanding that they are mutually dependent and equal. However, Sørensen and Torfing (2019a) regard the network and partnership structures in NPM as a hybrid democracy with the inherent tension between democratic leadership and democratic equality, that needs to be studied (Sørensen & Torfing, 2019b).

Research shows that the collaborations seem to take two forms: a conservative co-production form and a radical co-creation form (Røiseland & Lo, 2019). Co-production is mainly a collaboration between professional service providers and citizens as consumers and can also be found both in TPA and NPM. Citizens as *clients* co-produce in bureaucracies feeding the public sector with data needed to handle their case, and as *consumers* they co-produce services in schools, hospitals, etc. But these forms of participation are merely instrumental, and expert dominated within established institutional structures. In contrast to co-production, co-creation aims at being innovative and creating new organizations, procedures and services with results that better satisfy societal needs and purposes. Co-creations in networks challenge the established institutional structures and are a radical form of collaborations. In our opinion co-production in networks belongs to the Social Learning tradition, and co-creation belongs to the Social Mobilization tradition.

The Social Learning tradition and conservative New Public Governance

The Social Learning tradition (Friedmann, 1987) is concerned with learning through participation. Key questions are how to get people to participate in learning processes that contribute to opinion formation that can lead to a change in behaviour, and how to get dialogue between the rulers and the ruled. In this tradition, people's independent will and need for self-realization are emphasized and tried to be exploited within the framework of the state's authority.

Planning in this tradition demands that planning must include citizens in democratic processes. What characterizes these processes is the collective responsibility for the result, extensive dialogue between the participants and between the participants and various interest groups. One way to include citizens is through *negotiation planning*. Forester (1987, 1999) takes concrete planning conflicts as his starting point when he discusses negotiation planning. He shows that the planners can in practice be both negotiators and brokers, but in addition it will be required that the planners are spokespersons for weakly organized interests. Spokesperson or *advocate planning* is a common form of planning as a supplement to the traditional rational planning. In advocate planning (Davidoff, 1973) the governing authorities give weakly organized groups in local communities a spokesperson (advocate) to equalize their power with the actors representing the governing systems.

The Social Learning tradition seems to capture conservative NPG where communicative rationality and closed system view with focus on endogen factors dominate. This governing system is referred to as a self-grown structure. The organizational structure must free and expand individual action at the same time as it controls collective action. Organizational behaviour is sensible, collectively constructed and negotiated order. Change occurs through negotiation, conflict, mediation, compromise and mutual adaptation. For this governing system delivering *quality* in addition to *efficiency* and *effectiveness* is important (see Chapter 1). High quality means satisfying the needs and what people perceive as important to them but requires that the people are involved in the collaboration and manage to participate in both the formulation of the problems and the solutions to the problems. The participants become co-producers, and that the negotiation-based cooperation takes place between a limited number of actors, and within a given legal and economic framework defined by the sectors and units that the actors represent in the partnership. Challenges for successful collaboration are that the actors have different objectives, that the actors meet with limited mandates, or that the mandates are very unclear.

Potential conflicts in this governing system are between the service providers (with limited resources) and the service recipient (with unrealistic expectations). Such conflicts are often tried to be handled but can become unsolved because the government established economic and legal frameworks for cooperation are not challenged because the service providers regard themselves as servants of the top-down governing power and a conservative political ideology. When the actors are influenced and even limited by TPA and NPM from the units they represent, one cannot expect much new thinking and innovations from this governing system.

Summing up the tradition and presenting its public health politics

In the Social Learning tradition, planning is communicative in network organizations, and negotiation planning and spokesperson planning are highlighted. This planning tradition and governing system emphasizes increased quality in addition to increased efficiency and effectiveness (see Chapter 1). Delivering quality means satisfying people needs and for HiAP the aim for this governing system is to impose what is regarded as good for the people and to change their way of living. The tool is teaching people to make healthy choices and involving them learning by doing processes. The politics encompasses all sort of campaigns aimed at behaviour change such as quit smoking, drinking less alcohol, eat healthy food, be more physical active. However, individual behaviour changes are dependent on what matters and what one regards as quality of life. Planners must recognize that for some people smoking is regarded as an important and perceived quality, and a major weakness to this tradition and governing system is neglecting the counterforces in the environment and thus disregarding the structuring forces and determinants in the society that affect individuals, organizations and government. Actions are constrained from law and regulations, from the goal and result system, and from norms and culture, and even from professional standards (Synnevåg, Amdam & Fosse, 2019). As long as these structuring forces are regarded as given and even unchangeable in the negotiations, the institutional capacity of this governing system will stay weak. Thus, HiAP based on the learning tradition and the conservative form of NPG will not be able to mobilize people to take care of their health, and to form multi-actor collaborations with enough political power to change the determinants and structural forces that obstruct people from making healthy decisions and handle public health as wicked problem.

The Social Mobilization tradition and radical New Public Governance

The Social Mobilization tradition (Friedmann, 1987) differs from the first three traditions by emphasizing actions from below and changing the structural forces. The tradition focuses on capacity building and the promotion of new solutions that challenge established power structures. Participation from everyone is desirable to achieve learning, capacity building, new services and structural changes, and it is a prerequisite that everyone is regarded as equal citizens and that one recognizes to be mutually dependent on each other.

In planning according to the mobilization tradition, the actors have faith in collective mobilization and that collective actions can emerge in learning communities between the population and established governing powers. The *transactive planning* approach represents this tradition (Friedmann, 1973) and this planning emphasizes a broad grass-root mobilization to gain the strength to take greater responsibility for one's development and to influence the conditions under which one is working. In this planning process knowledge transforms into action through an uninterrupted sequence of relationships between people. Friedmann (1992) argues that knowledge and action can be linked through the process of critical understanding and radical practice, and that the planning process is a far-reaching learning process in which everyone can participate. Transactive planning can be illustrated as a learning spiral, see Figure 2.2. After a circuit in the spiral, one is back where one started, but with new knowledge and in a different situation. Levin (1988) refers to this as a process where it is usually individuals who go round the first circuit, and that they gradually get other individuals, groups and local communities to join them in the spiral of planning and practice. In the same way, Dryzek (1990) calls this process for an *inclusive democracy*, and Sager (1992) describes it as *integration of people and personal growth.*

Transactive planning focuses on how people's experiences can be used to shape policy. Transactive planning is based on the social mobilization tradition about the perception of the integration between knowledge and action, but nevertheless transactive planning stands in opposition to all three other traditions in that planning shall not be servile to the top-down power. Friedmann (1987) claims that transactive planning in society cannot be organized and supported by the power in the society but must grow from within the local communities. The planner who comes from outside can help to bring about a new self-understanding and make local communities skilled in self-help practices, direct action and negotiation, and create effective action programmes for structural changes. Planning shall be organized horizontally and directed from below and against the existing societal power. The planning is carried out in face-to-face dialogue with affected and interested parties, and planning process transforms knowledge into action through an unbroken sequence of interpersonal relationships.

The Social Mobilization tradition is dominated by communicative rationality and open system view with focus on exogen factors. In this tradition, the public sector units are perceived as one of many actors in a multi-actor system with competition to find niches where one can exist. Change occurs as natural evolution depending on changes in the environment, selection and power struggle to exist. Managers are expected to be innovative with an emphasis on securing their unit's existence. Following the mobilization tradition, governing of states is characterized by being a minimum state that takes care of the major national and global challenges and leaves other challenges to local and regional authorities as well as the voluntary and private sector.

In a similar way to the learning tradition, collaboration is organized in networks with the public, private and voluntary sectors and with free citizens as equal actors in network organizations, but in contrast to the learning tradition, this tradition focuses on co-creation and radical innovations to find new problem definitions and problem solutions, which are something more than the sum of the partners' traditional negotiating ways of working. The aim is to promote *efficiency*, *effectiveness*, *quality* and *legitimacy* by satisfying needs in society and to fulfil the purpose of the public sector with its core value such as democracy, equality, fairness and sustainable development.

What we call radical NPG is based on the Social Mobilization tradition. In this governing system, the network organizations themselves must build up the capacity and legitimacy to change the structures that define the network's room for action. This means that it is the process itself that must contribute to increasing their capacity and legitimacy. In this governing system, the state and the public are perceived as one of many actors in a multi-actor system and in competition to find niches to secure their existence. Knowledge and action must develop in critical and reflective localized processes, which increase one's own capacity for action to solve local problems, but also to promote demands for changes in the power structures. The actors are expected to be innovative with an emphasis on ensuring the existence of both their own organization and the network organizations in which they participated. However, NPG is a multi-actor collaboration involving people who represent TPA and NPM, and these governing systems do structure their behaviour and practice when it comes to understanding and solving problems. Laws and regulation, norms and standards, sector-thinking and unit-egoism make up this structuring force. But in contrast to the conservative form of NPG which regards the structural forces as untouchable, the radical form does confront these structuring forces to create and legitimate new political practice and structures.

Summing up the tradition and presenting its public health politics

Successful public politics in this tradition occurs when there is balance between top-down and bottom-up politics which legitimizes the democratic power that is exercised in the multi-actor collaborations. Reaching this balance in HiAP implies to mobilize people to take more responsibility for their own health and to put pressure on the structural forces in the society which determine public health and constraint people's possibilities to make healthy choices. In addition, it implies that the governing power structure allows this to happen so that a joint collective pressure from the top and the bottom can confront the established sector-thinking and unit-egoism and thus foster new and more holistic understanding of the situation and how to handle its problems. If these changes occur, there will be a new "normal" situation, hopefully with new and legitimated power balance between top and bottom.

The radical NPG represents the most complex and complete form of governing and accountability system. Its purpose is to increase efficiency, effectiveness, quality and legitimacy, and is thus especially relevant for multi-actor collaborations like HiAP where the democratic legitimacy and the capacity to act is depended on the process they can create.

Conclusion

In this chapter, we have identified four planning traditions and inherent governing systems that seem to be best suited in different situations, and we have discussed to which degree the four traditions are suited for Health in All Policies and for handling public health as a wicked problem. All the governing systems have problems with real involvement of inactive people, either they are perceived as a client, customer or citizen. The most powerful actors seem to achieve the most influence. We conclude that NPG, which is based on communicative logic and broad participation, is best suited for HiAP. But in modern societies the instrumental logic has dominated the communicative logic, making the practice of NPG with collaborative forms of planning challenging. NPG is proving to be particularly demanding to practice, since network-based collaborations involve actors from the dominating and fragmented government structure and require their support. The collaboration must produce output and outcome with high degree of efficiency, effectiveness, quality and fulfils the institutional purpose, and thus contribute to democratic legitimacy. Meeting this challenge requires reducing the tension between government and governance, and to set up thoughtful process designs that ensure good public participation, building individual and institutional capacity and democratic legitimacy. There is a need for changing the structural forces that hamper the public health work, and that is why we conclude that the radical form of NPG is needed to succeed with HiAP and the handling of public health as a wicked problem. Successful HiAP needs legitimated top-down power and bottom-up power in balance, and in the next chapter we discuss how radical NPG can be obtained using collaborative planning as will formation process. A crucial question is how one from above can support bottom-up mobilization when one can become the next target of structural changes?

References

Alexander, E. R. 2000. Rationality revisited: Planning paradigms in a post-postmodernist perspective. *Journal of Planning Education and Research*, 19: 242–256. https://doi.org/10.1177/0739456x0001900303

Allmendinger, P. 2009. *Planning Theory*. Houndmills, Basingstoke: Palgrave Macmillan.

Amdam, R. 2002. Sectorial versus territorial regional planning and development in Norway. *Journal of European Planning Studies*, 10 (1): 99–112. http://dx.doi.org/10.1080/09654310120099281

Arnstein, S. R. 1969. A ladder of citizen participation. *Journal of the American Institute of Planners*, 35 (4): 216–224. https://doi.org/10.1080/01944366908977225

Banfield, E. C. 1973. Ends and means in planning. In: Faludi, A. (ed.) *A Reader in Planning Theory*. Oxford: Pergamon Press.

Bolan, R. S. 1980. The practitioner as theorist. The phenomenology of the professional episode. *Journal of the American Planning Association*, 46 (3): 261–274. http://dx.doi.org/10.1080/01944368008977042

Bouckaert, G., Peters, G. & Verhoest, H. 2010. *The Coordination and Public Sector Organizations. Shifting Patterns of Public Management*. Houndmills Basingstoke: Palgrave Macmillan.

Bryson, J. M., Crosby, B. C. & Bloomberg, L. 2014. Public value governance: Moving beyond traditional public administration and new public management. *Public Administration Review*, 74 (4): 445–456. https://doi.org/10.1111/puar.12238

Bukve, O. 1997. *Kommunal forvaltning og planlegging*. Oslo: Det Norske Samlaget.

Christensen, T. & Lægreid, P. 2004. *The Fragmented State – The Challenges of Combining Efficiency, Institutional Norms and Democracy*. Working paper 3 – 2004. Bergen: Stein Rokkan Centre for Social Studies. https://norceresearch.brage.unit.no/norceresearch-xmlui/bitstream/handle/1956/1369/N03-04%5B1%5D.pdf

Christensen, T., Egeberg, M., Larsen, H. O., Lægreid, P. & Roness, P. G. 2002. *Forvaltning og politikk*. Oslo: Universitetsforlaget.

Christensen, T., Lægreid, P. & Rykkja, L. H. 2016. Organizing for crisis management: Building governance capacity and legitimacy. *Public Administration Review*, 76 (6): 887–97. https://doi.org/10.1111/puar.12558

Dahlgren, G. & Whitehead, M. 1991. Policies and strategies to promote social equity in health. Stockholm, Sweden: Institute for Futures Studies.

Davidoff, P. 1973. Advocacy and pluralism in planning behaviour. In: Faludi, A. (ed.) *A Reader in Planning Theory*. Oxford: Pergamon Press.

Davoudi, S. 2015. Planning as practice of knowing. *Planning Theory*, 14 (3): 316–331. https://doi.org/10.1177/1473095215575919

Dryzek, J. S. 1990. *Discursive Democracy. Politics, Policy, and Political Science*. Cambridge: Cambridge University Press.

Forester, J. 1987. Planning in the face of conflict: Negotiation and mediation strategies in local land use regulation. *Journal of the American Planning Association*, 53 (83): 303–314. https://doi.org/10.1080/01944368708976450

Forester, J. 1999. *The Deliberative Practitioner. Encouraging Participatory Planning Process*. Cambridge, Massachusetts: MIT Press.

Friedmann, J. 1973. *Retracing America. A Theory of Transactive Planning*. Garden City, New York: Anchor Press/Doubleday.

Friedmann, J. 1978. The epistemology of social practice: A critique of objective knowledge. *Theory and Society*, 6: 75–92. https://doi.org/10.1007/bf01566158

Friedmann, J. 1987. *Planning in the Public Domain. From Knowledge to Action*. Princeton NJ: Princeton University Press.

Friedmann, J. 1992. *Empowerment. The Politics of Alternative Development*. Cambridge MA and Oxford UK: Blackwell Publishers.

Giddens, A. 1984. *The Constitutions of Society: Outline of the Theory of Structuration*. Berkeley CA: University of California Press.
Hartley, J. 2005. Innovation in governance and public service: Past and present. *Public Money and Management*, 25 (1): 27–34. https://www.tandfonline.com/doi/abs/10.1111/j.1467-9302.2005.00447.x
Hartley, J., Sørensen, E. & Torfing, J., 2013. Collaborative innovation: A viable alternative to market competition and organizational entrepreneurship. *Public Administration Review*, 73: 821–830. https://doi.org/10.1111/puar.12136
Healey, P. 1997. *Collaborative Planning. Shaping Places in Fragmented Societies*. London: Macmillan Press.
Healey, P. 2003. Collaborative planning in perspective. *Planning Theory*, 2 (2): 101–123. https://doi.org/10.1177/14730952030022002
Healey, P., de Magalhaes, C. & Mandipour, A. 1999. Institutional Capacity-building, Urban Planning and Urban Regeneration Projects. In: Sotarauta, M. & Linnamaa, R. (eds.): Urban futures: A loss of shadows in the flowing spaces? *Futura*, 18 (3): 117–137.
Héritier, A. & Lehmkuhl, D. 2008. Introduction: The shadow of hierarchy and new modes of governance. *Journal of Public Policy*, 28 (19): 1–17. http://dx.doi.org/10.1017/S0143814X08000755
Hirschman, A. O. 1970. *Exit, Voice, and Loyalty: Responses to Decline in Firms, Organizations, and States*. Cambridge, MA: Harvard University Press.
Hood, C. C. 1991. A public management for all seasons? *Public Administration*, 69 (1): 3–19. https://doi.org/10.4236/oalib.1104579
Hood, C. & Dixon, R. 2015. *A Government That Worked Better and Cost Less? Evaluating Three Decades of Reform and Change in UK Central Government*. Oxford: Oxford University Press.
Innes, J. E. & Booher, D. E. 2004. Reframing public participation. Strategies for the 21st century. *Planning Theory and Practice*, 5 (4): 419–436. https://doi.org/10.1080/1464935042000293170
Langfield-Smith, K. & Smith, D. 2003. Management control systems and trust in outsourcing relationships. *Management Accounting Research*, 14: 281–307. https://doi.org/10.1016/S1044-5005(03)00046-5
Levin, M. 1988. *Lokal Mobilisering*. Institutt for industriell miljøforsking. Trondheim: SINTEF-Gruppen.
Lindblom, C. E. 1959. The science of 'muddling through. *Public Administration Review*, 19 (2): 79–88.
Osborne, S. P. 2009. *The New Public Governance? Emerging Perspectives on the Theory and Practice of Public Governance*. London: Routledge.
Pollitt, C. 2002. The new public management in international perspective – An analysis of impacts and effects. In: McLaughlin, K., Ferlie, E. & Osborne, S. P. (eds.) *New Public Management. Current Trends and Future Prospects*. London: Routledge.
Pollitt, C. & Bouckaert, G. 2000. *Public Management Reform: A Comparative Analysis – New Public Management, Governance, and the Neo-Weberian State*. Fourth edition. Oxford: Oxford University Press.
Putnam, R. D. 1993. *Making Democracy Work: Civic Traditions in Modern Italy*. Princeton, NJ: Princeton University Press.
Røiseland, A. & Lo, C. 2019. Samskaping – nyttig begrep for norske forskere og praktikere? *Norsk Samfunnsvitenskaplig Tidsskrift*, 35 (1): 51–58. https://doi.org/10.18261/issn.1504-2936-2019-01-03
Sager, T. 1992. Why plan? A multi-rationality foundation for planning. *Scandinavian Housing & Planning Research*, 9: 129–147. https://doi.org/10.1080/02815739208730300
Scharpf, F. W. 1999. *Governing in Europe: Effective and Democratic?* Oxford/New York: Oxford University Press.

Schön, D. A. 1983. *The Reflective Practitioner. How Professionals Think in Action*. London: Temple Smith.
Schön, D. A. 1986. Toward a new epistemology of practice. In: Checkoway, B. (ed.) *Strategic Perspectives of Planning Practice*. Lexington MA: Lexington Books.
Scott, W. R. 2002. *Organizations. Rational, Natural, and Open Systems*. 5th edition. London: Taylor and Francis.
Simon, H. A. 1957. *Administrative Man*. Second edition. Glencoe: Free Press.
Sørensen, E. & Torfing, J. 2012. Introduction. Collaborative innovation in public sector. *The Innovation Journal: The Public Sector Innovation Journal*, 18 (1): 1–14. https://innovation.cc/document/2012-17-1-1-introduction-collaborative-innovation-in-the-public-sector/
Sørensen, E. & Torfing, J. 2014. Enhancing social innovation through rethinking collaboration, leadership and public governance. In: Nicholls, A., Simon, J. & Gabriel, M. (eds). *New Frontiers in Social Innovation Research*: 145–169. Basingstoke: Palgrave Macmillan
Sørensen, E. & Torfing, J. 2019a. Interactive political leadership in theory and practice: How elected politicians may benefit from co-creating public value outcomes. *Administrative Science*, 9 (51): 2–18. https://doi:10.3390/admsci9030051
Sørensen, E. & Torfing, J. 2019b. Towards robust hybrid democracy in Scandinavian municipalities? *Scandinavian Political Studies*, 42 (1). 25–49. https://doi.org/10.1111/1467-9477.12134
Stoker, G. 1998. Governance as theory, five propositions. *Social Science Journal*, 50: 17–28. https://doi.org/10.1111/1468-2451.00106
Strand, T. 2001. *Ledelse, organisasjon og kultur*. Bergen: Fagbokforlaget.
Synnevåg, E. S., Amdam, R. & Fosse, E. M. 2019. Legitimising inter-sectoral public health policies: A challenge for professional identities? *International Journal of Integrated Care*, 19 (4): 1–10. https://doi.org/10.5334/ijic.4641
Torfing, J. 2016. *Collaborative Innovation in Public Sector*. Washington DC: Georgetown University Press.
Torfing, J., Sørensen, E. & Røiseland, A. 2016. Transforming the public sector into arena for co-creation: Barriers, drivers, benefits, and the way forward. *Administration and Society*, 51 (5): 795–825. https://doi.org/10.1177/0095399716680057
Zoete, P. R. 2000. *Towards Informal Levels in Urban and Regional Planning*. Paper at the 14th AESOP congress, 18–23 July 2000. Brno, Czech Republic.

3

COLLABORATIVE PLANNING AS A POLITICAL WILL FORMATION PROCESS WITH MOBILIZED CITIZENS IN PUBLIC SPHERES

The previous chapter showed that several governing systems can be used simultaneously in the management of societies and HiAP, but that radical New Public Governance is most suitable for HiAP. The governing systems have in common that they involve the exercise of legitimized political power. However, the purpose of radical New Public Governance is mobilizing political power to confront and transform the structuring forces that hamper solution to problems in accordance with the will of the citizens. This chapter discusses how the works of Habermas on theories of communicative actions have influenced governing and planning in societies, and how his political will formation process in public spheres can be adapted to collaborative planning and how the involved citizen must act in the process.

Introduction

The work of Habermas (1984, 1996, 1987) on communicative action theory have had a significant impact on several sciences, and with relevance to this chapter, we find a communicative turn from government to governance, and from instrumental to communicative planning, which can be linked to his works.

All governing systems are dependent on a political process that legitimizes the exercise of power and that gives the political actors the necessary power to act. Although all governing systems depend on such a political process, there is a sharp distinction between government and governance systems. In government, it is assumed that the various actors, through legislation and regulations and other inputs, have been assigned power and the capacity to act within their area of responsibility. In governance, the same actors must collaborate in network organizations, and their government power bases can become an obstacle to

DOI: 10.4324/9781003451273-3

defining joint problems and new solutions. Governance therefore depends on the top-down politics in government giving the collaboration the necessary political power, and the bottom-up communicative processes are a prerequisite for building network and partnerships between private, public and voluntary sectors, and between local, regional, national and international levels.

The communicative turn in planning represents a shift from instrumental planning to dialog, consensus and democracy and owes much to Habermas' theory of communicative actions. Communicative rationality emphasizes the meaning creating and action coordinating potential of the speech acts. Through discourses, the actors may arrive at common understandings of adequate actions, by which they feel bounded. Communicative rationality can contribute to building moral-forming communities, and to integrate individual and collective values, interests and needs.

In the planning literature, there is a growing understanding that the main challenge is not to choose between instrumental and the communicative planning and between top-down and bottom-up approaches, but how to integrate them in the practice. We recognize that the main challenge for HiAP and other governance network is to practice collaborative planning with the intention to increase the planning institution's capacity and legitimacy. The actors in this process are thrown between egoism and altruism, and between instrumental and communicative rationalities in political power structures. Thus, we argue that collaborative planning must regard planning as a democratic multi-actor process and work in a cross-sectoral and cross-level way internally, but also externally, to support the governance networks with acceptance, legitimacy and capacity to act. The actors must recognize that they are equal and mutually dependent on each other, they must conduct wisdom, and they must regard planning as a hybrid democratic process of knowing and doing.

The theory of communicative actions and the political will formation process

Modernization is usually associated with how society becomes more efficient and better able to produce goods and services by applying scientific techniques combined with organizational principles inspired by capitalist market economics. Critics of this instrumental modernization process point out consequences such as selfishness, fragmentation and loss of meaning (Habermas, 1984, 1987). It is also argued that the modernization of societies, with an emphasis on the introduction of new production technologies and new forms of governing, have led to professionalization and fragmentation, and to a greater distance between knowledge and action (Friedmann, 1992). Thus, in modern societies there is a risk that actions and patterns of action that give meaning to some persons, does not at all provide meaning to other persons because they lack the necessary knowledge both to be able to understand others' actions and for themselves to choose the right actions. This main feature of the modernization process is important to bear in mind when we discuss planning activities and their increased need for acceptance and legitimacy.

Habermas (1984, 1987) joins the general critics of the modern society. He claims that the positivist theory increases the distance between theory and practice, and that the formation of policy in modern society is fragmented and instrumental. Through his *theory of communicative action* Habermas tries to develop an extended universalistic concept of rationality, which not only covers instrumental rationality, but also communicative rationality (Habermas, 1996).

Habermas (1984, 1987) uses the terms *system* and *life world* to describe and analyse the modernization process. By system he means economic and political-administrative activity based on the steering, media, money, power and demands for results aiming at the goals of functional ability and effectiveness. This system is characterized by maximizing of individual benefit and instrumental rationality, and it can create *system integration.* In the life world, coordinated action builds on consensus created in ideal conversations. The focus is on the participants, and they are involved in communicative relations with each other. This results in a *social integration,* as opposed to system integration, and builds on a common evaluation of the situation, common goals and values, etc. The life world is tied to civil society and open, free, democratic processes in the public sphere.

Habermas (1984, 1987) claims that the system *colonizes* the life world, and that instrumental rationality thus displaces communicative rationality. As a counterweight to this development, he wants to strengthen the public sphere in society. By *public sphere* he means the social room created by actors acting communicatively. Thus, the public sphere does not become a separate institution or organization which one can study as structures, processes, norms, rules, etc. Public sphere is rather a network of communication and a process of interaction which assists in putting issues on the political agenda, ensures that solutions are passed and implemented, but also that the consequences are debated and evaluated. It is in the public sphere that moral judgements of what is fair, right, democratic, etc. will be expressed most clearly. One can thus claim that the public sphere represents the centre of democracy (Eriksen, 1994: 16), but it has to be added that the public sphere can be abused and manipulated, but it cannot be subjected to open pressure without the actors having to show themselves and so potentially weaken the force of their arguments and their legitimacy. The perspective here is that with the construction of the democratic constitutional state in a modern society, institutional arrangements for legitimizing this constitutional state have arisen. The line of reasoning is that no external authorities exist which guarantee the legitimacy of the democratic constitutional state; the state need to legitimize itself.

Habermas (1996) writes that institutions must secure their own legitimacy through *free processes of public will formation.* However, this public opinion-making process has little chance of being directly transformed into political action. The communicative power from the free opinion-making process in the political public sphere is through the passage of laws and regulations transformed into administrative power in the shape of state power to organize, sanction and implement. This means that it is not the individual morality of the actors, which decides the ability to act collectively and in solidarity, but rather the procedures for democratic will formation and collective decision-making which is institutionalized in modern societies. In this way, Habermas arrives at the normative point of view that a society should vitalize the connection between civil society and the political system through institutional reforms.

In the book *Facts and Norms*, Habermas (1996) meets the criticism against communicative rationality and the potential for consensus building. He does this by introducing several discourses with corresponding forms of rationality: *pragmatic benefit calculations*, *ethical-political*, *moral* and *juridical* discourses and formulates a model for political will formation process, which in our understanding can increase Scott's different forms of legitimacy (see Chapter 1):

- pragmatic discourses on benefit calculation and collective decisions on prioritization which can increase an institution's pragmatic legitimacy,
- ethical-political discourses about individual and collective identity and understanding of one's own ego, which can increase an institution's cognitive legitimacy,
- moral discourses about the extent to which positions in conflicts of interest can be generalized to fundamental values which can increase an institution's normative legitimacy, and
- juridical discourses where the social power in the initial discourses is transformed into laws and regulations and thus administrative power and can increase an institution's regulative legitimacy.

As we see, Habermas (1996) understands the political process as a will formation process starting with pragmatic discourses that further leads to ethical-political discourses and to moral discourses depending on the kinds of conflicts present. These discourses can lead to juridical discourses, which are oriented towards the consistence of laws and regulations. *Procedure-regulated negotiation* can be an alternative to discourses if they do not produce sufficient consensus (Figure 3.1).

Furthermore, he writes that negotiations are an alternative to discourses when there is no chance of agreement, but negotiations must be institutional arrangements or procedures that are accepted and legitimized. *Majority decisions* can be alternative processes when discourses and negotiations do not produce sufficient agreements. Habermas (1996) thus conveys that a legitimate decision does not necessarily reflect the will of everyone (consensus) but is the result of a democratic process. Discourses in the public sphere ensure democracy and create prerequisites for the legitimate exercise of power as a representation of the citizens' values and interests. It may be added that Habermas upholds that in a democracy, the majority will always be able to override the minority, but only if the process is accepted and legitimized.

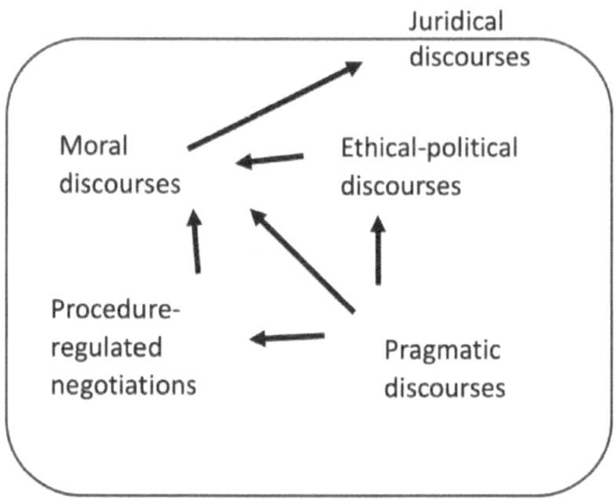

FIGURE 3.1 Discourses in a will formation and political legitimating process

Source: After Habermas (1996: 207) and Amdam (2010: 28).

In Habermas"theory of communicative action" a recurring line of argument is based on the *undistorted discourse* (Habermas, 1996) which is generally recognized as the ideal form of conversation to promote communicative rationality. From the work of Habermas (1984, 1987, 1996), one can draw the conditions for the undistorted discourse: All individuals who can speak and act are to be free to participate, free to question any proposal, free to make any proposal and free to express their attitudes, desires and needs. No speaker is to be hindered by force, either from inside or outside the discourse, from making use of these conditions. Actors who can through communicative processes, manage to create support for their opinions and actions, will be able to turn the social power into political power. Habermas argues that one cannot force communicative logic on the actors, and that consensus can only be realized to the extent that the discourse fulfils the demands to the process, namely *parity of power*, *the duty to argue* and *transparency or openness.*

Parity of power is important for the conversation to become a dialogue where the force of argument in the relationship between the actors decides the outcome of the conversation, not the power of one participant to forces views and norms on others. Parity of power implies that in the process the best argument shall be given the most weight, independent of who has the argument. Ideally, the strength of the arguments will decide what becomes regarded as important. For professionals, including planners, it may be difficult to accept and adapt to the parity of power demand, because they are trained as instrumental experts through their education. It is in situations in which knowledge is inadequate or diverse that it is important that professionals do not dominate and distort the ideal speech situation but participate in communicative discourses as equals together with lay people, elected officials and people from private and voluntary sectors.

Furthermore, the ideal conversation presupposes a public sphere and that the *duty to argue* applies even outside the discourse. This means that none of the actors are to execute any power in the discourse that makes any other actor become structurally subordinate, and that the weightiest argument ideally should be given the most weight in the process of making consensus. The duty to argue implies that whoever expresses oneself verbally will through the speech act communicate a connection to an *objective world* of existing facts and evidence, to a *subjective world* of personal experiences and emotions, and to a *social world* of accepted and valid norms. Thus, the instrumental rationality with focus on facts and evidence, meet the communicative rationality with focus on norms and experiences. It has to be added that facts and evidence are almost always depending on values, moral and views and that is why communicative rationality has to be made superior to the instrumental rationality (Dryzek, 1990; Friedmann, 1992; Habermas, 1996).

The listeners can evaluate how the statements relate to the *communicative validity claims*, that is that a speech act must be objective true, subjective sincere, normative right and comprehensible. If these validity claims are fulfilled, one may expect that communicative processes become meaningful and contribute to strengthening a shared understanding of problems and solutions, and thereby enhance anchoring, action, learning and legitimacy. If not, the actors in the communicative process will undermine their own acceptance and legitimacy, and who wants to do that?

The demand for reason together with the demand for openness and transparency, force the participants to defend their statements towards citizens that are formal parts in the discourses. The participants and the public must have similar options to contradict what is said by means of a new speech act, and the actors will thus become involved in a process with a mutual duty to give arguments for one's statements in a public sphere.

Regarding public health, it must be mentioned that Scambler (2001a) has edited a book about Habermas, critical theory and health, which we value as a major contribution to the understanding of the fundamental challenges in public health work. In the introduction chapter to the book, Scrambler writes an overview of Habermas"voluminous production, and he discusses central terms in Habermas" contribution to the development of critical theory. The overview consist of terms like system, life world, public sphere, rationality, legitimation crises and of course the theory of communicative action, and Scambler tries to relate these terms to the public health work (Scambler, 2001b). However, ideal conversations and policy legitimating processes are not an easy way to create a collective will (Jacobsson, 1997). But in societies and communities which are based on democratic values, the communicative action theory is the main approach to legitimating politics, laws and plans. Democracy and transparency are the best guarantee against illegitimate execution of power.

The communicative turn in governance

The concept of governance has gained widespread currency across many of the social sciences, and many disciplines have struggled to analyse the broad set of changes in the relationship between state, market and civil society; the conceptual trinity which has tended to dominate mainstream analysis of modern societies. In the concept of governance, actors and institutions attempt to establish a capacity to act by blending their resources, skills and purposes into a viable partnership. The governance concept points to the creation of new structures that is a result of the interaction of different actors. Governance has become necessary because of the restructuring of the state and has been reflected in several ways, such as:

- a relative decline in the role of formal government in the management of social and economic relationships,
- the involvement of non-governmental actors in a range of state functions at a variety of spatial levels,
- a change from hierarchical forms of government structures to more flexible forms of partnership and networking,
- a shift from provision by formal government structures to sharing of responsibilities and service provision between the state and civil society, and
- the devolution and decentralization of formal governmental responsibility to regional and local governments (United Nations, 2009: 73).

Governance is always an interactive process because no single actor, public or private, has the knowledge and resource capacity to tackle problems unilaterally. In contrast to government's silos, governance is to be regarded as a network with loose structural connections where cooperation between independent but mutually dependent actors leads to dialogue-based cooperation and consensus solutions. For example, Rhodes (1997) refers to governance as a form of governing where public, private and voluntary actors, through network cooperation and partnership building, work together to find answers to common challenges in the political-administrative governing system. He highlights four characteristic features of governance:

- Mutual dependence between organizations. Governance is broader than government and includes non-governmental actors.
- The need to exchange resources and negotiate objectives entails repeated interaction between network members.
- The game-like negotiations between the network members are based on trust and regulated by fixed rules of the game that have been agreed upon.
- Networks are not accountable to the state, they are self-organized. The state's borders are changing and the borders between public, private and voluntary organizations are shifting and opaque. The state can still manage the network in an indirect and imperfect way (Rhodes, 1997: 4).

However, governance is criticized: Recognizing the power dependence in collective actions implies accepting that intentions do not always match outcomes

(Stoker, 1998: 22), the governance's co-ordination process has been characterized rather neatly as "managing a nobody-in-charge world" (Stoker, 1997), and there is warnings that the growing obsession with governance mechanisms as a solution to *market failure* or *state failure* should not lead us to neglect the possibility of *governance failure*. One must avoid seeing governance as necessarily being a more efficient solution to problems of economic or political co-ordination than markets or states. Failures of leadership, differences in time scale and horizons among key partners, and the depth of social conflicts can all provide the seed for governance failures (Stoker, 1998: 24). One must ask critical questions about the new governance institutions that emerge and supplement the government institutions (Jessop, 1997), and for example does Swyngedouw (2005) discuss the *Janus face* of governance, and concludes that instead of enhanced democracy, extension of "holder" participation and improved transparency, governance can become élite technocracy and power-based interest intermediation and face considerable internal and external problems with respect to accountability and legitimacy.

According to Olsen (1988), organizations in government and governance are institutions defined as a structure between the individual and society. The structure is not a neutral mirror of micro-motives or macro-force but modifies and is modified by both forces. The structure manages authority and power, but also collective wisdom, ethics and norms, and shows the signs of a certain political order (March & Olsen, 1976). Institutions create order in behaviour and ways of thinking, but they are still temporary and limited forms of order. Political institutions are part of the political process, and, over time, the institution itself will exercise a conservative power by defining which actors, problems, solutions and deciding factors which are to be recognized as legitimate. The political institutions can be separated from community and society and become a sort of filter between the organization and its context. It is therefore important that the political institutions are subject to a completely open public scrutiny so that citizens can monitor what the institutions are doing. The separation of political institutions from community and society can only be counteracted by a strengthening of democracy and transparency through media coverage, open hearings, public meetings, etc. Here we see the importance of what Habermas describes as the *public sphere* (Habermas, 1984, 1987) and political will formation (Habermas, 1996). When citizens meet to discuss collectively relevant questions or to act together, they develop a communicative power that can and should exert influence on the political system.

The communicative turn in planning

Instrumental rationality can justify the public sector with technically and economically efficient production of goods and services (input and output legitimacy), but like Habermas, Eriksen (1993) claims that this is not enough for the public sector. The public sector's legitimacy must also be based on communicative rationality, which means that the process through communicative rationality contributes to making the public sector more democratic, transparent, accountable, fair and humane (outcome legitimacy). The legitimation process can be top-down or bottom-up, or a combination. Top-down legitimacy gives the public sector responsibility and power to administer laws, regulations, resources and other tools for public production. Legitimacy from below depends on how well a political institution can stimulate collective actions and build capacity (empowerment) (Healey, de Magalhaes & Mandipour, 1999).

Communicative planning is rooted in the interaction of social life, and is oriented towards inter subjective understanding, the co-ordination of actions through discussion, and the socialization of members of the community. Communicative planning regards legitimacy, discourses, participation, action and learning as key issues. The planning process shall serve to build up social, institutional and political capacity, which can become a new local and regional institutional resource and political power. Healey (1997: 314) calls this a *soft infrastructure* (governance), but without attention to the *hard infrastructure* represented by the formal policy structure (government), it will be difficult to change the current policy. These formal systems are often seen as immovable constraints that simply are just "there". However, these constraints are never fixed, they are socially constructed, and they can be reconstructed through dialog, mobilization and learning and using social, political, and administrative power.

In instrumental planning one assumes that the formal power of the planning unit is made legitimate through laws and regulations, applicable norms and values and the hierarchy of authority. In communicative planning, on the other hand, one assumes that it is the planning process itself that will give the planning unit and the plan legitimacy and the needed acceptance, anchoring, support and participation. Instrumental rationality tells us how to combine the means to achieve given ends and is appropriate for goal-oriented behaviour within a means-end structured problem area. Instrumental planning can lead to bigger local and regional dependency on external institutions and forces. According to Stöhr (1990) it can also weaken the local communities' capability to learn and to handle challenges.

When the state has a strong role as a major developer of the society and communities, the government institutions have the legitimacy to conduct instrumental and mainly top-down master planning. This form of planning is fitted to solve many of the problems the planning is facing as far as one is talking about the forming of governmental top-down and sectorized public services providing. However, planning is not just about forming policies and programmes, but also about implementing these through changing norms and creating collective actions. A common critique of instrumental top-down planning is that neither the plan nor the implementation is embedded in the local and regional institutions. The plans are usually drawn up by experts and without broad participation. The bottom-up planning, as an alternative approach to traditional top-down planning, places the emphasis on direct democracy, autonomy in the decision-making of territorially organized communities, local self-reliance and experiential social learning. Its starting point is the locality, because the civil society is most readily mobilized around local issues. Civil society is the many-standard order that arises from those values and interests which are shared by most of the people in particular communities. The aim is to mobilize the civil society and transfer the social power to political power.

In planning it can be fruitful to separate sectoral planning from territorial planning (Amdam, 2005, 2022, 2010). The *sectoral planning* is an integrated part of the top-down nation building process and the government structure, and is regarded as legitimate when it provides technical and economic effects seen from the different sectors. For the *territorial planning*, the situation is different. This is mainly a bottom-up institution building process based on social mobilizing and governance. In many ways, territorial planning will come to oppose and challenge the sectoral planning and power, but the territorial planning will not generate more legitimacy and capacity than the process itself can create and the sectorized national authorities want to give the planning. Thus, the territorial planning representing the governance, becomes very dependent on the acceptance from the national state authorities, and consequently, it is important that the planner not only has knowledge of planning as a tool, but also knows the political reality in which the tool is to be used. Planners who lack the necessary insight in the political structure, culture and processes can make mistakes that can lead both the planner and the planning into a state of discredit.

The instrumental form of planning is criticized for being based on cause-and-effect relationships that are not real (not evidence-based), for being expert-dominated and for being oppressive. Communicative planning, on the other hand, is criticized for placing too much emphasis on achieving consensus, for being time-consuming and for not taking sufficient account of structuring forces in the environment. This means that regardless of how one positions oneself, the planning can be criticized. This dispute between instrumental and communicative planning happens even though several scientists (Friedmann, 1992; Habermas, 1996) which examine the fundamental challenges in modern society, claim that the biggest challenge now is to combine instrumental and communicative rationalities, both in theory and in practice. Communicative rationality cannot totally replace instrumental rationality; it can only restrict the latter to a subordinate domain (Habermas, 1996).

From the perspective of instrumental logic, it is assumed that the planning institution has enough legitimate power to decide the direction, put problems on the agenda, make decisions and implement them. The planning institution can define what is relevant knowledge, and it has the power to translate that knowledge into actions. Used in areas where a planning institution has both the power and the will to implement a plan, instrumental planning can be an effective way of linking knowledge to action. From the perspective of communicative logic, on the other side, it is recognized that different institutions have power, and that there are countless structures and forces, so that the planning process must provide the plan and the planning institution with acceptance, legitimacy and the power to implement the plan. Healey (2003, 2009), Forester (1987) and Innes and Booher (2015) all argue that communicative planning must to a larger extent consider instrumental and structural forces, and that the collaborative process, with a combination of instrumental and communicative planning, can help build and change institutions and challenge the structural forces.

Many scientists have participated in the debate about collaborative planning, and they have helped to clarify the differences between instrumental and communicative planning and rationality (Healey, 2003, 2009; Forester, 2012; Davoudi, 2015). In the article *Turning point for planning theory? Overcoming dividing discourses*, Innes and Booher (2015) take this debate somewhat further and portray collaborative planning as a relation between actors and structures. The argument is that insofar as people have created these institutions, people can also change them. They write that "...collaborative rationality is an adaption from idea of communicative rationality to real-world practice of collaborative policy making with stakeholders" (Innes & Booher, 2015: 15).

We interpret these authors' contributions to the discussion of collaborative planning as arguments for building on communicative planning, but at the same time provide room for instrumental, expert-driven planning in a democratic planning process that can both challenge and change institutional powers. Thus, collaborative planning is regarded as an intermediate form of planning. Communicative planning and collaborative planning have many common characteristics, but the former is more theoretically oriented, and the latter more oriented towards real-life problems and to translating the theory into practice. Collaborative planning is typically used in situations in which the division of responsibility is unclear at the starting point, and in which stakeholders are mutually dependent on each other and need to trust each other and to cooperate. The planners and the participants are equal and cannot command each other, but by creating conditions that will bring stakeholders together, the planning process can help them practice wisdom and build collective capacity and learn so that they can recognize the situation and develop new practices. In a collaborative planning process, one needs to engage oneself together with others in a collective learning process that will increase the collective ability to make use of information and to handle conflicts.

Collaborative planning focuses the relations between the actors involved and the context as structural forces with private, public and civil institutions. Collaborative planning is not just about finding new ways to move forward, but also a matter of building acceptance, legitimacy and the capacity to handle new challenges. In collaborative planning, one needs to recognize that there is not a single best solution that can be worked out, but that there may be many solutions that will at least be improvements compared to an unsatisfactory status quo state.

Transforming communicative action theory to planning practice

Undoubtedly, Habermas's work (see especially Habermas, 1996: *Facts and Norms*) on communicative action theory has had a major influence on government and planning. But Habermas' work is regarded as normative, ideal and theoretical, and has been criticized for not treating power in political processes as a reality. Foucault is often regarded as representing the other extreme, compared to Habermas. Foucault (see e.g. Foucault, 1980) is known for his analyses of power, which contributed to understanding and explaining power in political processes, but he is criticized for not paying attention to how to turn knowledge into action. The criticisms of Habermas and Foucault are not entirely without merit, but should, according to Flyvbjerg and Richardson (2002), be nuanced: Habermas writes about power and how democratic political power can become legitimate rule of law, and Foucault understands power as a condition to change repressive power relations in a democratic way. Well-known authors in planning theory have positioned themselves to Habermas and Foucault in different ways.

The Habermas-oriented collaborative planning position is particularly linked to Patsy Healey, Judith Innes and John Forester. They focus on the planning's context and legitimacy, how planning can contribute to local and regional capacity building, and how to legitimize institutions that can advance local and regional policies (Healey, 1997; Innes & Booher, 2010). In addition to the theory of communicative rationality, collaborative planning also includes theories of urban development, institutions, complexity and not the least, relations between actors and structures. This is evident when Healey, in the preface to the book *Collaborative planning: Shaping places in fragmented societies*, writes that through collaborative planning political communities can organize themselves to improve the qualities of a city (Healey, 1997: xii). Her starting point is that modern societies are fragmented, and that they need planning that strengthens consensus and collaboration between public, private and voluntary organizations. Healey (2003) maintains that she builds on Habermas's work, but that she relies at least as much on Giddens's concept of structuring (Giddens, 1984). Forester (1999) takes a pragmatic perspective on planning as *deliberative* process and leans heavily on Habermas while being inspired by Foucault. He takes note of what planners really do in practice.

The more Foucault-based position deals with the so-called dark side of planning, and includes work by, among others, Flyvbjerg (1991a, 1991b), Flyvbjerg and Richardson (2002) and Hillier (2002, 2003). Through their work, they show that consensus-oriented policy formulation based on communicative theory, despite good intentions, is vulnerable to the weight of tactics in the form of manipulation, control, confusion and exclusion. Whereas Flyvbjerg mentions *antagonistic* conflicts between actors without respect for others, Hillier tries to bring such antagonistic conflicts into what is called *agonism*, where actors can be in conflict but have basic respect for each other. Conflict is here seen as something positive and constructive, and something that is important to a planning process. Hillier

(2002) differentiates between associative and agonistic democracy, and states that people who do not participate in formal, inclusive democratic planning processes can nevertheless, through informal processes, influence planning and policy by ignoring, exiting and participating in networks, lobbying shareholders, engaging in direct actions etc. Hillier concludes that participative planning processes have their "insiders" and "outsiders", and that it is utopian to believe that planning should include everyone in formal consensus-building processes. Planners should therefore acknowledge that planning has a dark side, and rather than overlook and hide conflicts, they should help bring such conflicts to light and to an agonistic state in which, through negotiation and mediation, one can agree to disagree yet find solutions one can live with.

In planning and politics actors in power can define how a situation should be viewed, as well as how problems should be defined and solved instrumentally. However, investigations of political processes often show that the processes can be viewed as illogical and unprofessional. In plain text, this means that politics often has a logic that professionals and planners are not aware of (Flyvbjerg, 1996). In all political processes actors can act tactically in relation to each other to gain special advantages, which might take the form of misinforming, holding back information, making promises they do not intend to keep, etc. Such power plays are part of the political process, and planning must take them into account (Forester, 1987). Communicative planning is based on the presumption that the present and the future are being formed in inter-subjective learning processes between actors, and the planner becomes one of many actors contributing to the process. Thus, most people will see the planner and the other participants in the planning process as political actors with their own values, needs and interests (Flyvbjerg, 1996, 1998).

We regard planning as policymaking, and politics can be seen as an activity that evolves around finding ways of formulating problems, trying to get these formulations accepted as binding and eventually organize continuous problem-solving activities around these problems (Jacobsen, 1964). Thus, both politics and planning evolve around having the power to promote wishes, interests and values. However, great uncertainty about the future due to the complexity and the pace of change in modern society, has led to a lack of trust in rational calculations as a model of decision, and has moved the attention over to models that are based on communication and learning (Sager, 1990). This change also affects the view of planning and leads to essential changes in the relationship between planning and politics. In instrumental planning models based on rational calculations, it is in theory possible to separate politics and planning. Thus, planning can be separated to a subject-independent activity based on preparing political decisions, but if one accept that planning and politics can be divided, one can easily fall into the trap of seeing planning as something positive because one believes that it is logical and functional. In addition, one can see politics as something negative because one sees it as illogical and dysfunctional (Minogue, 1993: 20). That does, however, not mean that politics *is* illogical. In situations where there is a lack of evidence-based knowledge and academically supported solutions, or at least a lack of solutions that provide meaningfulness for all people, politicians as elected representatives must make decisions because the problem must have a solution, and the consequence of a non-decision might be worse. Solutions arrived at to such problems can be symbolic or real.

In our opinion the *transactive planning* model (Friedmann, 1973) comes closest to describe planning as a political will formation process. Transactive planning focuses on how people's experience can be used to form policy. The planning is not carried out by experts for the object of the plan, but in face-to-face dialogue between those involved and interested. Personal growth and joint action are the key elements in this planning, and planning is not divorced from other social action in which the aim is to gain control over social processes that effect one's welfare. Transactive planning use democratic processes to encourage opposition to the established authorities and can in some situations result in changes in the political power and policymaking. Such mobilization can start with individuals and be expanded to movement and gain strong political power, but that these movements can gradually lose their basis for existence because they have managed to put the issues they are fighting for on the political agenda, and made a desired solutions part of the production of the established governing system.

The need for wisdom in collaborative planning

Democratically and politically active citizens who engage in conscious problem-solving are central characteristics of transformative planning and radical New Public Governance. The purpose of participation is to involve the people in competence building so that they can handle their own and society's problems to a greater extent. When these actors enter face-to-face discourse, the premises are at least implicit:

- that the actors are interested in developing a common understanding and to negotiate with each other,
- that they are free and equal, and potentially equally competent,
- that everyone must admit mistakes and change their minds when confronted with a better argument, and
- that everyone acts authentically and truthfully towards each other.

The requirement for all who participated in the face-to-face dialogue is to maintain the linguistic validity requirements for ideal conversations that what one says must be objective true, subjective sincere, normative right and comprehensible. In these conversations, the actors' knowledge, attitudes, opinions and actions are challenged by others, and one is forced to argue for one's position and actions. In this way, the transformative planning, with a combination of instrumental and communicative logic, can contribute to reflection, learning and thus to a new understanding of the problem and what are possible solutions, and can thus also contribute to both individual competence building and collective capacity building (Amdam, 2020).

This competence building planning and governing corresponds to the understanding of collaborative planning that, for example, Simin Davoudi has. She writes that planning should be perceived as a critical and reflective learning process where the actors should show wisdom towards each other when they discuss the central elements of planning, namely actions and the questions about *why* changes are desirable and necessary (knowing to what end), about *what* changes are important, and about *how* to proceed to change (Davoudi, 2015). She argues that planning should shift focus away from a planning based on evidence, to a planning informed by evidence, and shift from regarding knowledge as something that planners have, to knowing as something planners do. She argues that rather than focusing on *knowledge* one should look at planning as a *practice of knowing and learning*. She does not deny the utility of objective knowledge in planning, but she does point out that "...planning as practice of knowing is multidimensional; it is situated and provisional, collective and distributed, purposive and pragmatic, and mediated and contested" (Davoudi, 2015: 328). In this way, she states that planning takes place in a process with many different actors seeking benefits within structural forces. Over time, this process where the actors seek to fulfil their interests and maximize benefits becomes new structural forces with institutional characteristics such as defined knowledge, established values and norms, and, not the least, legislative regulations. Therefore, participants in collaborative planning should exercise wisdom (phronesis) as practical judgement based on a critical reflective process that combines:

- *knowing why* (moral choices),
- *knowing what* (theories and concepts),
- *knowing how* (crafts and skills), and
- *doing* (actions) (Davoudi, 2015: 321)

In Amdam (2020), we have discussed how this critical reflective process can be linked to the social practice epistemology (Friedmann, 1978) and different form of legitimacy (Scott, 2014), and how the process may increase the network's capacity and legitimacy through a reflective learning process focusing on the actors' practical judgement and planning as the practice of knowing. See Figure 3.2.

- The vertical line represents instrumental rationality and is linked mainly to regulative and pragmatic legitimacy. The horizontal line represents communicative rationality and is mainly linked to normative and cognitive legitimacy. A more equal combination of the two rationalities in collaborative processes is needed in modern societies.

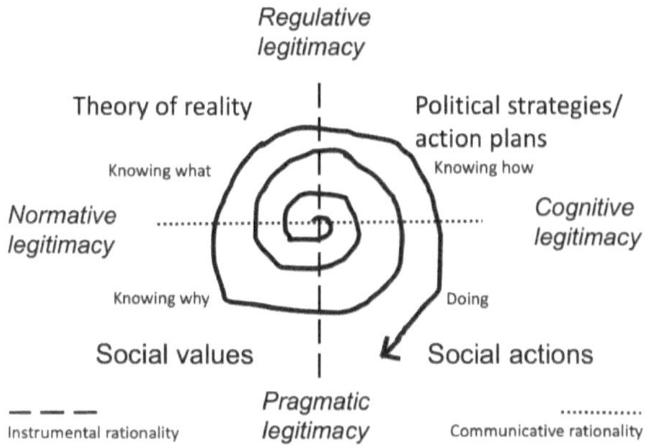

FIGURE 3.2 Co-creation and the spiral of citizen participation

Source: Based on Amdam (2020: 44).

- The four sections represent Davoudi's categories *knowing why*, *what*, *how* and *doing*, and Friedmann's similar categories *social values*, *theory of reality*, *political strategies and social action.*
- The co-creation spiral represents *spiral of citizen participation*, the collaborative learning process as the practice of knowing (Davoudi, 2015) aimed at enhancing the collaborative network's institutional capacity and legitimacy.
- The spiral also illustrates that Habermas` political will formation process with the different discourses that take place in the four sections with relations to both instrumental and communicative forms of rationalities at the same time.

The doings – pragmatic discourse about social actions related to cognitive and pragmatic legitimacy

The doings are handled in pragmatical discourses about social actions. Social actions are created in an intersection between instrumental cost–benefit calculations and cultures characterized by cognitive models. Over time, these patterns of action can form cultures with some form of orthodoxy including professional standards and organizational traditions, which can hinder collaborative co-creation (Synnevåg, Amdam & Fosse, 2017, 2019). Thus, instrumental and communicative rationalities meet in pragmatic discourses, and it is reasonable to claim that implementing actions with high degree of pragmatic and cognitive legitimacy is a prerequisite for achieving the other forms of legitimacy in the will formation process. If the actions are considered practically useless and different from the orthodoxy, the basis for strong institutional legitimacy and capacity may vanish. Actions that are regarded as useful for people, units and organizations can be a strong motivational force for people to participate in network processes, but in a network organization where actors find that the benefits are small in proportion to costs, conflicts of interests can easily arise.

The relevance to HiAP is clear. In HiAP there is a need for facts and evidence verifying that healthy living such as increased physical activity and reduced consumption of alcohol and unhealthy food, quitting smoking, etc. have a positive health effect for both for individual and societal level. However, the research is often contested by the industry that makes the products. In addition, even if the products are proved to be unhealthy, the use of them is heavily influences by tradition and culture which can be difficult to change. People's unhealthy way of living can be considered useful for them self, even when documented that the activities heavily burden the public sector health budgets.

Knowing how – ethical-political discourses about political strategies/ detailed plan for action related to regulative and cognitive legitimacy

Knowing how is about choosing tactics that are regarded as appropriate ways to proceed to obtain desired change. The tactics for solving problems and meeting challenges have both a regulatory and a cognitive dimension and is an ethical-political discourse about who's interest to prioritize. These detailed plans for action must remain within the instrumental legal and economical regulatory framework, but these regulatory constraints on the plans must be balanced against the cognitive models which are established patterns and professional standards of action that over time form cultures with a form of orthodoxy.

In collaborative processes, one can easily predict that every new planned action will meet some resistance based on cognitive models of how problems can and should be understood and handled, and on different interpretations of laws and regulations.

For HiAP the knowing how-discourses are well known from coordinating the use of economic, physical and personal resources. A redesign of cities to make them healthier and more sustainable can serve as a typical example. This redesign process demands giving priority to some groups of people on the cost of other groups, for instance prioritize young people and pedestrians higher than car drivers, will normally generate conflicts between the involved groups and can represent a discontinuity of traditions. Another example is giving priority to non-smoker by banning smoking in public places.

Knowing what – moral discourse about theories of reality related to normative and regulative legitimacy

The knowing what-discourse is about what matters for the citizens and for the community and is often expressed with visions and strategies for handling the most important challenges. However, knowledge about the situation is always limited and contested and can be regarded as a moral discourse. Knowledge of actual legislation, regulations and other instrumental regulative documents form an important part of the theories of reality. In addition, objective and evidence-based knowledge is often regarded as instrumental facts in the same way as knowledge of legislation and regulations. But only evidence-based knowledge, which is independent of time and space, can be regarded as objective and value neutral. All other types of knowledge are based on values, either implicitly or explicitly. In planning practice much of the knowledge will be based on actors' subjective perceptions, which are largely influenced by social values. In this process, there will be conflicts between the different professions and disciplines' normative and regulative-based arguments. Furthermore, there will be a dilemma between how the experts' objective facts and evidence-based knowledge should be emphasized in relation to lay people's more experience-based knowledge. Therefore, it is important when deciding what matters that many and different actors can contribute to the process of developing as much common understanding of the situation and the internal and external challenges as possible.

For HiAP this discourse is about giving priority to public health issues on the political agenda in competition with many other precious issues like regional and local economic development, public services to children at schools, and to elderly people at nursing institutions. The political agendas are changing constantly due to unexpected events, competing interest groups, changed political power etc. Keeping HiAP high on the political agenda is an enduring communicative process with arguments based on facts and norms. One example here is the discussion on banning smoking at homes and in cars with children, which in Norway is halted because many people regrade this banning for intervening too much in the private sphere.

Knowing why – a juridical discourse about social values related to pragmatic and normative legitimacy with strong regulative implications

Knowing why represents the juridical discourse in the political will formation process and is about core values in the society. In juridical discourses the social power in the initial discourses is transformed into laws, regulations, plan, documents and other administrative power. In politics and planning social values are expressed by missions and porous in the text of laws and regulations and they are important to all actors' interpretations of a situation, solutions they can accept and the actions that are considered useful. However, altruistic social norms and values are challenged from the instrumental egoistic calculation of what is useful for oneself. Thus, juridical discourses are related to normative and pragmatic legitimacy. This means that for the systematic planning in organizations and networks, all activities, effects and consequences are assessed against values such as democracy, sustainability, equality and against the satisfaction of individual needs.

For HiAP this is a very important, enduring and challenging discourse. In this debate WHO is an important international political force with strong arguments in support of HiAP which is commonly accepted among politicians and made a regulative norm for nation's public health policy. However, when it comes to the realization of the policy, HiAP as a multi-actor collaboration approach to public health, struggle with sector- and unit-egoism and lack of collaboration. This is well documented in Chapters 1 and 2.

The complexity of wisdom and lack of practical judgement in HiAP

The discussion above on how collaborative processes can increase legitimacy and capacity, shows that the multitude of actors in the interactive network process face several structural forces that can reduce the actors' acceptance and the network's legitimacy. This situation is challenging for all the representatives involved because they are supposed to conduct wisdom in a position constrained by sometimes conflicting regulative, normative, cognitive and pragmatic structural forces from the network and from the organization they represent. However, if the participants in the network regard planning as the practice of knowing, and through a mutual learning process can conduct wisdom and practical judgement, there is a potential to build political institutions with legitimacy and capacity. To conduct wisdom in this complex situation, demands that the involved actors participate as *whole persons* in the discourses and expose their values, knowledge, skills and capability to implement for criticism in all the discourses in the will formation process. In this way they can build individual competence and collective capacity.

Communication helps create meaning related to what is correct and right, and to reveal power structures. Innes and Booher (2015: 8) draw on the work of Castells (2009) and claim that power relations are created and maintained through communication and that rules, norms, values and practices are shaped in communicative networks. This is how public, private and civil organizations become institutionalized and come to constitute structuring forces in society. Planning has a potential to change these institutions if the communicative processes manage to contribute to new understanding among key stakeholders and the public. We must remember that when actors have been able to create structuring political institutions, they can also change them. Thus, we must advance the question to what extant HiAP functions as political will formation process, which we do in Chapters 4, 5 and 6.

Conclusion

The communicative action theory has influenced the practice of governing and planning, and forced HiAP to become a radical New Public Governance practice that can increase HiAP's institutional capacity and democratic legitimacy. We consider Habermas's work on discursive will formation as a flexible and promising guide to this future institutional reform of HiAP. In his work, he argues in favour of combining instrumental and communicative rationality in an open opinion and will formation process (Habermas, 1996). In this process Habermas presents different discourses with their respective rationalities, and together they form a political legitimating and capacity building process. It is through public debate among free citizens that proposals can be justified, but for the citizen to conduct wisdom in the political will formation process, is a prerequisite. In this chapter we have discussed how this political will formation process can be adapted to planning as a process of knowing. This is a process seeing planning as a collaborative learning process where the participants, through reflection and action in the most ideal conversations possible, challenge each other's actions, values, knowledge and skills and in that way contribute to making each other wiser and more competent. This makes planning a continuous process were showing wisdom about why, what, how and doing, and in the next chapter we discuss the design of a collaborative planning as political will formation process, and the planner's role as a process manager.

References

Amdam, R. 2005. *Planlegging Som Handling*. Oslo: Universitetsforlaget.

Amdam, R. 2010. *Planning in Health Promotion Work: an Empowerment Model*. Abingdon, Oxon and New York: Routledge.

Amdam, R. 2020. Planning and innovation in a collaborative framework. In: Hagen, A. & Higdem, U. (eds.) *Innovation in Public Planning. Calculate, Communicate and Innovate*. Cham, Switzerland: Palgrave Macmillan.

Amdam, R. 2022. *Samskapt berekraft. Ei modell for samarbeidsdriven planlegging og innovasjon*. Rapport - nr. 115/2022. Volda: Høgskulen i Volda. https://bravo.hivolda.no/hivolda-xmlui/handle/11250/2991502

Castells, M. 2009. *Communication Power*. Oxford: Oxford University Press.

Davoudi, S. 2015. Planning as practice of knowing. *Planning Theory*, 14 (3): 316–331. https://doi.org/10.1177/1473095215575919

Dryzek, J. S. 1990. *Discursive Democracy. Politics, Policy, and Political Science*. Cambridge: Cambridge University Press.

Eriksen, E. O. 1994. *Politikk og offentlighet. En introduksjon til Jürgen Habermas' politiske teori*. LOS-senter Notat 9405. Bergen: Norsk senter for forskning i ledelse, organisasjon & styring.

Eriksen, E. O. 1993. *Den offentlige dimensjonen*. Verdier og styring i offentlig sektor. Tromsø/Bergen: Tano Aschehoug.

Flyvbjerg, B. 1991a. *Rationalitet og Magt. Bind 1. Det konkretes videnskab*. København: Akademisk Forlag.

Flyvbjerg, B. 1991b. *Rationalitet og Magt. Bind 2. Et Case-baseret studie av planlæging politikk og modernitet*. København: Akademisk Forlag.

Flyvbjerg, B. 1998. *Rationality and Power. Democracy in Action*. Chicago: University of Chicago Press.

Flyvbjerg, B. 1996. The dark side of planning: 'rationality and realrationalitat'. In: Mandelbaum, S. J. et al. (eds.) *Explorations in Planning Theory*. Rutgers: Centre for Urban Policy Research.

Flyvbjerg, B. & Richardson, T. 2002. Planning and Foucault. In search of the dark side of planning theory. In: Allmendinger, P. & Tewdwr-Jones, M. (eds.) *Planning Futures. New Directions for Planning Theory*. Abingdon and New York: Routledge.

Forester, J. 1987. Planning in the face of conflict: Negotiation and mediation strategies in local land use regulation. *Journal of the American Planning Association*, 53 (83): 303–314. https://doi.org/10.1080/01944368708976450

Forester, J. 1999. *The Deliberative Practitioner. Encouraging Participatory Planning Process*. Cambridge, Massachusetts, MA: MIT Press.

Forester, J. 2012. On the theory and practice of critical pragmatism: Deliberative practice and creative negotiations. *Planning Theory*, 12 (1): 5–22. https://doi.org/10.1177/1473095212448750
Foucault, M. 1980. Power/Knowledge: Selected Interviews and Other Writings, 1972–1977 (Colin Gordon ed.). New York: Pantheon.
Friedmann, J. 1973. *Retracing America. A Theory of Transactive Planning*. Garden City, New York: Anchor Press/Doubleday.
Friedmann, J. 1978. The epistemology of social practice: A critique of objective knowledge. *Theory and Society*, 6: 75–92. https://doi.org/10.1007/bf01566158
Friedmann, J. 1992. *Empowerment. The Politics of Alternative Development*. Cambridge MA and Oxford UK: Blackwell Publishers.
Giddens, A. 1984. *The Constitutions of Society: Outline of the Theory of Structuration*. Berkeley CA: University of California Press.
Habermas, J. 1984. *The Theory of Communicative Action. Volume 1: Reason and the Rationalization of Society*. London: Heinemann.
Habermas, J. 1987. *The Theory of Communicative Action. Volume 2: Lifeworld and System: A Critique of Functionalist Reason*. Boston, MA: Beacon Press.
Habermas, J. 1996. *Between Facts and Norms: Contributions to a Discourse Theory of Law and Democracy*. Massachusetts and London: MIT Press.
Healey, P. 1997. *Collaborative Planning. Shaping Places in Fragmented Societies*. London: Macmillan Press.
Healey, P. 2003. Collaborative planning in perspective. *Planning Theory*, 2 (2): 101–123. https://doi.org/10.1177/14730952030022002
Healey, P. 2009. The pragmatic tradition in planning thought. *Journal of Planning Education and Research*, 28 (3): 277–292. https://doi.org/10.1177/0739456x08325175
Healey, P., de Magalhaes, C. & Mandipour, A. 1999. Institutional Capacity-building, Urban Planning and Urban Regeneration Projects. In: Sotarauta, M. & Linnamaa, R. (eds.) Urban futures: A loss of shadows in the flowing spaces? *Futura*, 18 (3): 117–137.
Hillier, J. 2002. Direct action and agonism in democratic planning practice. In: Allmendinger, P. & Tewdwr-Jones, M. (eds.) *Planning Futures. New Directions for Planning Theory*. Abingdon and New York: Routledge.
Hillier, J. 2003. Agonizing over the consensus: Why Habermasian ideals cannot be real. *Planning Theory*, 2 (1): 37–59. https://doi.org/10.1177/1473095203002001005
Innes, J. E. & Booher, D. E. 2010. *Planning With Complexity. An Introduction to Collaborative Rationality for Public Policy*. London: Routledge.
Innes, J. E. & Booher, D. E. 2015. A turning point for planning theory? Overcoming dividing discourses. *Planning Theory*, 14 (2): 195–213. https://doi.org/10.1177/1473095213519356
Jacobsen, K. D. 1964. *Teknisk hjelp og politisk struktur*. Oslo: Universitetsforlaget.
Jacobsson, K. 1997. Discursive will formation and the question of legitimacy in European politics. *Scandinavian Political Studies*, 20 (1): 69–90.
Jessop, B. 1997. A neo-Gramscian approach to the regulation of urban regimes: Accumulation strategies, hegemonic projects, and governance. In: Lauria, M. (ed.) *Reconstructing Urban Regime Theory: Regulating Urban Politics in a Global Economy*: 51–73. London: Sage.
March, J. G. & Olsen, J. P. (eds.). 1976. *Ambiguity and Choice in Organizations*. Bergen: Universitetsforlaget.
Minogue, M. 1993. Theory and practice in public policy and administration. In: Hill, M. (ed.) *The Policy Process. A Reader*. London: Harvester Wheatsheaf.
Olsen, J. P. 1988. *Administrative Reforms and Theories of Organization*. Notat 88/31. Bergen: LOS-senteret.
Rhodes, R. A. W. 1997. *Understanding Governance. Policy Networks, Governance, Reflexivity and Accountability*. Buckingham, Philadelphia: Open University Press.

Sager, T. 1990. *Communicate or Calculate. Planning Theory and Social Science Concepts in a Contingency Perspective*. NORDPLAN Dissertation 11. Stockholm: Nordic Institute for Studies in Urban and Regional Planning.
Scambler, G. (ed.). 2001a. *Habermas, Critical Theory and Health*. Florence, KY, USA: Routledge.
Scambler, G. 2001b. Unfolding themes of an incomplete project. In: *Habermas, Critical Theory and Health*. Florence, KY, USA: Routledge.
Scott, W. R. 2014. *Institutions and Organizations: Ideas, Interests, and Identities*. 4th edition. Sage Publications.
Stöhr, W. 1990. Synthesis, introduction and on the theory and practice of local development in Europe. In: Stöhr, W. (ed.) *Global Challenge and Local Response*. London and New York: Mansell.
Stoker, G. 1997. Public-private partnership and urban governance. In: Stoker, G. (ed.) *Partners in Urban Governance: European and American Experience*. London: Macmillan.
Stoker, G. 1998. Governance as theory, five propositions. *Social Science Journal*, 50: 17–28. https://doi.org/10.1111/1468-2451.00106
Swyngedouw, E. 2005. Governance innovation and the citizen: The Janus face of governance-beyond-the-state. *Urban Studies*, 42 (11): 1191–2006. https://doi.org/10.1080/00420980500279869
Synnevåg, E. S., Amdam, R. & Fosse, E. M. 2017. Public health terminology: Hindrance to a health in all policies approach? *Scandinavian Journal of Public Health*, 46 (1): 68–73. https://doi.org/10.1177/1403494817729921
Synnevåg, E. S., Amdam, R. & Fosse, E. M. 2019. Legitimising inter-sectoral public health policies: A challenge for professional identities? *International Journal of Integrated Care*, 19 (4): 1–10. https://doi.org/10.5334/ijic.4641
United Nations. 2009. *Planning Sustainable Cities. Global Report on Human Settlements*. United Nations Human Settlements Programme. London: Sterling: Earthscan.

4

THE ISTOL-MODEL, A COLLABORATIVE PLANNING DESIGN

The conclusion in Chapter 3 was that HiAP to gain democratic legitimacy and institutional capacity within the radical New Public Governance regime, must be organized as a political will formation process with several discourses. The discussion in this chapter is about how the theoretically grounded work of Habermas on a political will formation process with juridical, moral, ethical/political and pragmatic discourses, can be adapted to a planning model with institutional, strategic, tactical and operative planning, and that is designed to stimulate development processes consisting of the variables context, mobilization, organization and implementation. The term ISTOL is an abbreviation from the first letter of the word institutional, strategic, tactical, operative and learning.

Introduction

In several works, we have adapted Habermas' model of political will formation to a model for regional and local planning and development, see Amdam (1997, 2001, 2005, 2010, 2020, 2021, 2022). The model is based on a link between discourses in policy legitimating processes (Figure 3.2), variables in collaborative development processes (Figure 4.1) and tools in collaborative planning (Figure 4.2). The model is designed to achieve increased institutional capacity for action and democratic legitimacy through identifying which development variables must be influenced, and to find planning tools that can influence the variables in the desired direction. We sum up the existing research by claiming that regional and local planning approach with the tools: institutional, strategic, tactical and operative planning, combined with a monitoring and evaluation processes seem to be a good concept for stimulating the variables in local and regional development: context, mobilizing,

DOI: 10.4324/9781003451273-4

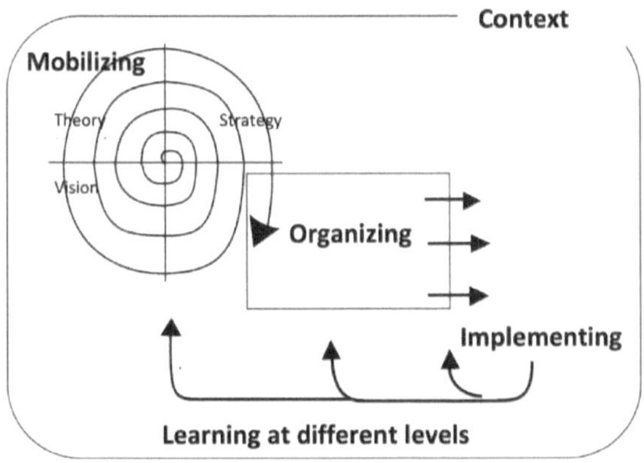

FIGURE 4.1 Variables in collaborative development

Source: Amdam (2010: 55).

organizing, implementing and learning. Furthermore, the planning tools and the development variables are linked together in political will formation and political institution building processes.

By using the well-known terms institutional, strategic, tactical and operative that exist in both planning and management, we get to convey that planning and management are closely linked, and that planning can be a tool for leadership and steering. Another strength of the model is that it emphasizes the relationship between internal and external political power. Actors can, by advocating for their values, interests, and needs, alter the structural power that has been integrated into the system over time, including presumptions, action patterns, routines, and rules. In addition, the

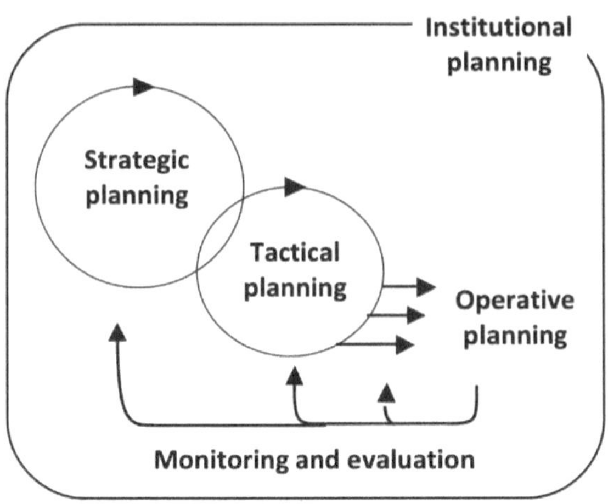

FIGURE 4.2 Tools in collaborative planning

Source: Amdam (2010: 56).

structural power can influence and socialize actors trying to achieve changes. Consequently, the model also gives an illustration of power not being a fixed variable, but subject to changes in both time and space. In this way, the actors in the process become aware of their society and their organization's dependence on the environment and the actors' often limited opportunities to get something done on their own.

Variables in collaborative development processes

So far, we concluded that HiAP is a process of building legitim institutional capacity in communities. Political strong local and regional communities are often characterized by people participating in both professional and local networks, and by the integration of local horizontal and global vertical relationships. Community with a strong civil society and a strong democratic process is the main key to a dynamic local and regional development; see among others Dryzek (1990), Stöhr (1990), Friedmann (1992), Bennett and McCoshan (1993), Putnam (1993), Forester (1993) and Storper (1997).

In the field of planning science, Patsy Healey (1999) has presented a model of *institutional capacity building* in communities as a continuing process with *knowledge resources*, *relations resources* and *mobilization capability* which together summarize to the institutional capacity. The knowledge and relation resources are in her model regarded as prerequisites for the mobilization capacity, and they all together form the strength of the institutional capacity. She maintains the importance for communities to have a strong local institutional capacity to response to external forces and the internal development, but the capacity will differ from community to community and from time to time. A weakness of this model is that institutional capacity primarily seems to be regarded as an endogen process, and the model is unclear on how exogenous processes form the institutional capacity.

Labonte and Laverack (2001a, 2001b) have delivered central work on capacity building in health promotion. Labonte and Laverack (2001a: 112) write that capacity in health promotion often is presumed to exist as an unproblematic resource that can be monitored and measured. However, more rigorous works describe capacity as social and organizational relations with dynamic qualities rather than static properties. They have identified nine domains in a community capacity building process, and according to Labonte and Laverack (2001a: 130) these nine domains must combine the logic of health promotion top-down programmes with bottom-up mobilization and emancipation to:

- improve community participation,
- develop local leadership,
- build empowering organizational structures,
- increase community members' problem assessment capacities,
- enhance community members' ability to "ask why",
- improve community resource mobilization,

- strengthen community links to other organizations and people,
- create an equitable relationship with outside agents, and
- increase community control over programme management.

We agree that the domains are important, but in our view, they need to be included in a more structured and operative model. We have identified five critical factors which we call variables because the strength of them differs over time and from place to place, and as far as we have experienced, in successful capacity building all of them must have a minimum strength (see Figure 4.1).

The variables are context, mobilizing, organizing, implementing and learning. All the variables in the model mutually affect each other. They can add up to both positive and negative self-reinforcing processes. Our experience suggests that a capacity building process requires that all four internal variables are reasonably strong, and that the context variable does not promote or constrain these variables too strongly. We believe that, on the one hand, planning should be mobilizing in relation to promoting new recognitions, new organizational methods, new actions and stimulating learning. But on the other hand, planning should also be controlling and allocative in relation to a sensible use of natural resources, capital and people. We would like to clarify, that satisfying the four internal variables in development processes is a necessary, but not a sufficient condition for a successful process. Therefore, it is precisely the interaction between the external macro forces in the environment and the internal forces locally and regionally that is decisive for the overall result. This interaction can of course lead to greater local and regional imbalance in that the skilled and strong local and regional communities achieve the most, and the less skilled and weak communities become losers. Too strong a dosage of national policy can create dependency, and too weak a dosage can create local and regional differences. A constructive top-down policy is perceived as necessary to promote bottom-up policy, but a good balance is not easy to achieve in practice. Our experience is that such processes can be stimulated with the help of planning as tools if the planning process manages to stimulate the relevant variables and at the same time contributes to a good balance between them.

Tools in collaborative planning processes

There is no planning tool that is appropriate in all situations, and therefore is it important that the planners not only have knowledge of planning as an activity, but that they also know the political reality in which the tool is to be used. Jacobsen (1964) has given a definition of politics which is widely used, and which is very useful in this context. He writes that politics can be understood as an activity that consists of formulating issues, trying to get the issues accepted as binding and possibly organizing continuous problem-solving activities around them. In comparison, Lundquist (1976) has defined planning as a future-oriented process where the actors seek to gain control over their surroundings to thereby be able to carry out their intentions. A similar definition is given by Østerud (1979: 12), who writes that community planning is a system of strategic decisions to design future courses of action. These definitions express much the same, namely that politics and planning include putting problems on the political agenda, gaining control or power and influencing the production of the problem solution. When one perceives planning as a political process, the challenge is to create an acknowledgement so that the current problem is accepted, and to organize actions so that the problem is solved in a future-oriented and intended way. Thus, politics and planning are about the power to promote one's own and others' wishes, interests and values.

When setting up a planning system, it is logical to start from Parsons' (1977) system theory and the perception that social systems are made up of four subsystems: the pattern-maintaining subsystem, the integrating subsystem, the political subsystem and the economic subsystem. Alexander (2000) takes this system theory as a starting point and discusses how different forms of rationalities in planning are associated with different approaches to planning. He divides planning approaches into four paradigms: planning as frame setting, communicative practice, coordinative planning and rational planning (Alexander, 2000: 247). He argues that the different approaches and methods can and should be used in different situations, but also together.

Bringing these contributions into a planning process, we have found similarities between Alexander's four paradigms, Friedmann's social practice epistemology with the categories *social values*, *theory of reality*, *political strategies and social action*, and with Davoudi's planning as the practice of knowing with the categories *knowing why*, *what*, *how* and *doing*. In our opinion these system theory-generated elements can be expressed with the terms: institutional, strategic, tactical and operative planning which are more commonly used in practice. See Figure 4.2.

Variables and tools brought together in the political will formation process

As we have written above, we consider Habermas's work on discursive will formation a flexible and promising guide to future institutional reforms and enforcing governance. In our understanding of Habermas's political will formation or legitimating process the *juridical discourse* concerns the rules of juridical consistency. This is planning as a systematic process of developing a frame of reference for future planning and decisions. These issues concern the relation between the context and the planning institution, and the legal influence of the formally decided planning documents and other juridical norms. This discourse is about the mission, capacity and legitimacy, and is the topic of what we call *institutional planning* and *knowing why*.

The *moral discourse* concerns the conflicts of norms and values, and is a topic for mainly communicative planning, that is planning as a social interactive process between actors who are seeking consensus and mutual understanding. These are questions which are the issues for mobilizing and for *strategic planning* and *knowing what*.

The *ethical-political discourse* involves a discussion of whose needs; interests and values are to be favoured. Conflicts of interests that are often connected with the utilization of resources in coordinative planning, that is planning with the focus on how to deploy organizations to undertake the necessary actions at the appropriate time to accomplish mutual agreed upon outcomes. This discourse refers to the questions of organization, coordination and *tactical planning* and *knowing how*.

The *pragmatic discourse* concerns the discussion of facts and data and is a discourse tied mainly to instrumental rationality, that is planning as a deliberative activity of problem-solving, involving rational choices by self-interested individuals or homogeneous social units. The objective of rational planning is for the actors to decide to what ends future actions should be undertaken, and what course of action would be most effective. These elements are at the core of implementation and the *operative planning* and the *doing*.

Knowing why – frame setting, institutional planning and partnership

In Chapter 3 we concluded that knowing why in planning is a juridical discourse about social values related to pragmatic and normative legitimacy with strong regulative implications. The juridical discourses concern the legitimacy of the governing body itself and the consistency of the legal rules. The results of juridical discourses depend on the consensus obtained in the other discourses in the will formation process, or the negotiated agreement and majority decisions. A successful political will formation process creates laws and regulations which are guidelines for governing the society and with implications for which activity that shall hold regulative, normative, cognitive and pragmatic legitimacy.

We interpret the juridical discourse to be the formal treatment and the status of the planning document that the planning and development process creates, but also as the plan for the planning process. We call this institutional planning, and by that we mean the framework for the activity that is set by the higher government level, and the framework that the planning unit itself has set. Thus, the juridical discourse can be where a planning activity ends and the plan is given a formal status defining why, what and how to implement further actions, and even regulates how lack of doing and wrongdoing shall be sanctioned. The discourse can also be the frame setting starting point for a new planning process, for instance a project plan for HiAP in regional and local communities. In relation to Luke's (1974) different forms of power, this means having power to design the planning process.

In many contexts, local and regional development work is included in national and international programmes, and then the programme itself will form a framework for how the development work can be carried out. Furthermore, the local and regional actors' own plans and guidelines will also act as frameworks for the development work. Institutional planning is about planning the planning process, or meta-planning and meta-governance when it comes to the management of network organizations where the responsibility for the actions is divided between many organizations and between government levels.

When development work is organized as programmes and projects, there is a need for partnerships between the actors, but the establishment of these partnerships requires that the actors can commit themselves to the partnerships. We will use *institutional partnerships* as a term for these partnerships, and by this we mean judicially binding agreements that regulate the responsibilities between the actors for implementing the programme or project. Institutional partnership is highly formalized, has an external given acceptance and legitimacy, and a limited number of members. The main purpose of these partnerships is frame setting for other partnerships and processes. *Institutional planning* is the process of establishing these partnerships and the frame of reference for future decisions.

Institutional planning is concerning the relation between the planning unit and the context and is what Alexander (2000) calls "planning as frame setting". This planning emphasizes the need in planning to set a framework for the planning activity. Such frameworks can be previous binding decisions and existing understanding models and frameworks that have a governing effect on thoughts and actions. Essentially the institutional planning concerns the relations between the community and the structural powers in the context that create both opportunities and obstacles for the local and regional communities as political actors. In our works, we emphasize the mutual relations between them in line with Giddens (1984). In concrete terms, that means that the building up of an institutional capacity in a region or local community takes place in interaction with the surroundings. Therefore, the planning must attempt to bring to light structural forces in the context and find out to what extent they represent opportunities or threats for the community. Furthermore, one must look at the power in the planning process and to what extent the process transforms people's values, interests and actions. This means that actor-structure relations also become important for the other discourses in Habermas' model of political will formation.

We usually organize the planning and development effort in regional and local communities as a project with a steering group as the coordinating body, and we often set up a team for teaching, supervising and evaluation (Amdam, 2011, 2022, 2021). The main purpose for the project is to set up a planning that stimulates mobilizing, organizing, implementing and learning processes in the community, and to produce plan documents with institutional, strategical, tactical, operative and evaluating content. But the local process will usually not give the process and plan sufficient legitimacy. There will be a need for formal decisions in several institutions in the superior political power structure. Local and regional planning exist in the interface between actors from both the vertical and horizontal power structure, the different actors are in the special situation of needing approval and legitimacy from both structures. That is, from the governing levels; municipality, county and state and from the governing systems; voluntary, private and public sectors including democratically elected representatives. In practical planning this implies that the planning process must incorporate actors from both the horizontal and vertical structure, and that the planning documents must be formally accepted in the appropriate organizations that belong to the two structures.

It is important to emphasize that regional and local planning can be intensified by way of a project, but that it is none the less a continuous process. Organizing planning and development work as a project can be a useful method of approach when an all-out effort is required for a limited period in a limited area. A well-established project presupposes that the members of the steering group have arrived at a reasonable degree of agreement about aims and means, and not least about the limits of and the mandate for the project. Without the clarification of such questions, internal conflicts within the steering group can well paralyze the whole project. It is also vital that the participants as far as possible enjoy equal rights when it comes to the terms of participation.

Summary – criteria for institutional planning and partnerships

Below we have summarized our requirements for HiAP as a planning and development work that aims to stimulate regional and local capacity building at institutional level.

Requirements for planning documents:

- HiAP should be based on a plan for the development work. This plan should, as a minimum, describe the background, purpose, working method, milestones and framework for the planning process, and it should say something about special themes, interests, groups, etc. which must have special weight.
- HiAP that is carried out as a project should have a project plan that states what the aim of the project is, how the project is planned to be led and managed, how the interdisciplinary and coordinated efforts of several people and organizations are planned to be carried out, what the project's time and cost frameworks are, and last, but not least, how this one-off task is to be integrated into the different partnership organizations' routines and carried forward after the project period.

Requirements for HiAP planning process:

- HiAP should be based on juridical discourses between local, regional and national levels of government and between the private, public and voluntary sectors and reflected in institutional partnership agreements.

- There should be an appropriate balance between management from above and management from below, so that the process promotes increased mastery/capability at all levels.
- Special procedural steps should be taken to include weakly organized interests and groups.
- HiAP should have a four-dimensional view of power which means power to design and setting frames for the public health work, and to keep the partners accountable for their activity and lack of activity in HiAP.
- The project/process management must have the competence to see the process from the outside and to intervene the weakest variables of the development process at any time.

HiAP as institutional planning should contribute to:

- Increase the capacity to design the HiAP work and the regulative legitimacy of the local and regional planning documents, so that they achieve status in relation to legal documents and other planning documents.
- Increase HiAP's capacity to design the process and the regulative legitimacy of HiAP.
- Increase the delegation of power and responsibility from the vertical governance structure to local and regional political institutions and clarify the division of labour between local and central government.
- Increase the legitimacy and acceptance of democratic local and regional political institutions which include representatives from the public, private and voluntary sectors (partnerships), which monitor and analyse local regional development and which have the legitimacy and power to introduce the necessary measures to promote the desired development.

Knowing what – mobilizing, strategic planning and partnership

In Chapter 3 we concluded that knowing what is a moral discourse about theories of reality related to normative and regulative legitimacy. Moral discourses concern different values and associated patterns of action that are opposed to each other. The moral discourse concerns the question of what is important to people and is linked to people's actions, needs, interests, and values within what one can call the good society. Moral discourses in planning are a process to mobilize broad participation, and the content of the strategic planning should reflect the level of recognition the participants are at. Where the recognition of the development trend and the challenges is weak and scattered, it can take a long time to mobilize people to change the situation.

By the mobilization variable we mean activating and gathering of the people to promote collective and individual actions. This can be stimulated by strengthening common perceptions about development trends and challenges, and about how one can work to reach common goals. This means that locally and regionally one can focus on structures and processes, on connections between the local community and society at large, and on how local and regional governing bodies can work to influence these elements and relationships. A strong mobilization variable in local and regional development means basically that there exists a realistic understanding of the present situation and of the future, and that there is a reasonable measure of agreement about to how to act to achieve the desired future. Strategic planning may be used as a tool to stimulate the acquiring of knowledge, to increase awareness and to bring about a new understanding in the hope that individuals, organizations and communities can change their behaviour and their situation.

The mobilization is dependent on *strategic partnerships* which are little formalized and have a relatively flat hierarchy. The activity is variable, and the number of members is changing. These partnerships are often mobilized around a core of members when the situation demands it, and there is a need for a great number of members to influence the agenda setting. The partnerships need members that share a common understanding of the situation and a common vision of the future and agreed upon strategies. In these partnerships the partners from the government structure will clearly experience dilemmas when participating in governance structures, because much of the strategic work in governance partnerships is to influence the government's public sector political agenda.

Strategic planning can be understood as what Alexander calls "communicative planning". Planning as a communicative practice sees planning as a social interactive process where the argumentation brings about common understandings and cooperation. This activity can also be called a consensus-building activity (Innes et al, 1994; Healey, 1997), and can involve developing a broadly shared understanding of development trends and challenges, visions for what kind of situation one wants and strategies to reach this situation. This means that one gathers around a political agenda (Lukes, 1974) and builds up a collective capacity to influence the political understanding of what matter in the community.

Strategic planning refers to fundamental questions such as what is typical for the situation with its development characteristics and challenges, what sort of future do we want, where should we start and how can we make changes to move from the present situation in the direction of the ideal. The purpose of strategic planning is to orient oneself in relation to one's own situation, the environment and the future, and on this basis to formulate a vision and point out areas of effort and strategies to reach this desired state. Issues like this touch on ideological values that can be expected to be stable over a period. It is however a moot point to what degree planning alone can manage to change such standpoints.

Creating support for the use of one's own comparative advantages is important in the mobilization work. We have experienced that to achieve this, it is important to engage in opinion-breaking processes that bring together the population and other important actors across political government levels, government systems and political interests and across personal characteristics such as age, gender, profession, status, etc. (Amdam, 1995). In this way, group formations, organization-building, alliances and networks can be stimulated which can generate a local social power which can eventually be transformed into a political power. Experience shows that social power can be stimulated, but that the process can take time before it mobilizes enough power to achieve major political changes. Nevertheless, it seems to be quite clear that a successful mobilization process can provide sufficient new recognition of the weaknesses of the current situation to bring about comprehensive changes in the other variables (Amdam, 2011).

One important experience from our involvement in strategic planning is that people easily get mobilized in the discussion of strategic issues that concern them, but in the political will formation process there is a critical stage between the discussion and the actual involvement in organization that can implement actions. Some people seem to be more interested in talking about what other must do, than taking responsibility of getting something done. It is nevertheless the case that, through mobilizing and communicative planning, various actors can develop a common value base and perceptions about key development trends and challenges.

Summary – criteria for strategic planning and partnerships

As a summary of the discussion in this chapter, we highlight the following requirements that HiAP as a strategic, mobilizing and political agenda-setting process must fulfil.

Requirements for document content:

- Strengths and weaknesses in the current situation must be clarified, opportunities and threats in the future must be assessed and a vision of the desired future situation must be formulated.
- The focus must be on important areas of effort and strategies to bring the community from the current situation to the desired future situation.
- Each strategy should be described with background, needs and what one specifically wants to achieve as a result. Furthermore, each strategy should be mentioned with a description of cooperation and organization, costs and financing, expected bottlenecks and ways to handle them, expected positive and negative consequences of the strategic action and proposals for specific projects, measures and activities.

Requirements for the HiAP planning process:

- HiAP as a planning process should handle value conflicts and promote consensus on value prioritizing in moral discourses. National overall prioritized areas of effort should be discussed, and one must prioritize what are the most important areas of effort at regional and local level.

- HiAP should promote integration and personal growth aimed at individual and collective self-understanding.
- HiAP should have a three-dimensional view of power and the input side of policy production, which means putting important areas of effort on the political agenda.
- The process management should have competence to mobilize and motivate participation, identify problems, set the agenda, etc.

HiAP as strategic planning should contribute to:

- Increase HiAP's capacity to put on the political agenda and the normative legitimacy of HiAP.
- Reduce the extent and intensity of value conflicts and promote a common recognition of development features and challenges in the current situation and a common support for a vision that expresses the desired future situation.
- Stimulate local and regional political power, personal growth, sense of community, flexibility, strong local identity and self-confidence combined with an accepted responsibility for one's own situation.
- Mobilize civil society as a moral-forming community by stimulating an active voluntary sector.
- Strengthen the alliance between the voluntary sector and public authorities to transform the local social power into political power.
- Promote a social atmosphere that can have a stimulating effect on individual and collective actors.

Knowing how – organizing, tactical planning and partnerships

Getting from mobilization to implementation always involves some form of organization of the resources needed. By the organizing variable we refer to the fact that power can form new organizations and changes in temporary and permanent organizations, and thus increase the institutional capacity. In this process of organizing the process is about using own competence, creativity, motivation, raw materials, capital, technology, etc., in the best possible way to satisfy needs.

We have defined knowing how as an ethical-political discourse about tactics or procedure related to regulative and cognitive legitimacy (see Chapter 3). The political/ethic discourse relates to the questions of organization and coordination, which are issues for tactical and coordinative planning. Tactical planning is what Alexander calls "coordinative planning". In a politically fragmented societies, it will often be decisive for the society's further development that organized cooperation is achieved across established organizational boundaries. The knowing how process in planning deals with the conflicts of interest that often relate to the utilization of resources. It is therefore vital to achieve a division of labour and partnership with voluntary associations and organizations, private enterprise, public administration and politicians. It may be an ideal to seek to achieve harmony between local organizations and their surroundings, but in practice conflicts are unavoidable, simply because the organizations must fight for limited resources between different and often irreconcilable needs, interests and values.

These conflicts are right at the core of the *tactical planning* whose aim is to obtain and deploy resources among responsible actors. Planning as coordination involves creating regulations, guidelines, organizations, etc. which promotes coordinated actions. The tactical planning gets its framework from the strategic planning through the choice of the area of efforts (strategies). The tactical planning includes acquiring, developing and organizing the resources. Tactical planning focuses on the dimensioning of the resources and the distribution between different sub-areas, sectors, local communities, programmes, etc. In relation to dimensions of power, this form of planning applies to having the authority to make decisions, or to prevent decisions being made (Lukes, 1974). In contrast to the planning at the strategic level, the planning at the tactical level is focused on the short-term resource effort to achieve the strategic goals, it is more detailed and implementation-oriented, and it is not only indicative, but it is binding.

Tactical planning is usually a conflict-filled arena where visions for the community and the various actors' benefit calculations and self-interests meet; an arena where the communicative and instrumental logics stand particularly strongly against each other. The focus is on how to deploy organizations to undertake the necessary actions at the appropriate time to accomplish mutually agreed upon outcomes. This involves giving priority to activities over a period in the form of a *programme of action.* These programmes organize and prioritize defined projects, activities and changes. Normally organizations have scant resources at their disposal and are very dependent on other actors to get things done, but lack of responsibility and accountability is a main challenge in the implementation of local and regional multi-actor action programmes. Therefore, it is very important when these actions programme are set up, that each collaborating organization takes responsibility for their part of the actions.

Collaborative action programmes can stimulate producing of realistic ideas about what the organizations are able to achieve, alone and in *tactical partnerships*. These partnerships are highly formalized, have a limited number of members, and have a strong need for an agreed upon and accepted common action programmes. In addition, the partners need to get their part of the common action programmes prioritized in their own action programmes. Thus, the partners are caught in situation of uncertainty. How much can they contribute to the common action programme, and how much involvement are their own organizations willing to accept. If there is a big difference between what the partners say they shall do, and what they do, they will lose trust and become less important partners in the future.

Regarding HiAP, the responsibility for implementation may lie with public, private or voluntary organizations, therefore it is desirable and necessary to have partnership agreements. Tactical partnerships are very much about finding solutions between the visionary and wishful thinking (strategic planning) and the realistic and practical (operative planning). If HiAP's tactical planning is to be real, the actors must agree to the partnership's action programme and the relevant projects included in it. The various members must make a concrete commitment to contribute resources in the form of work and capital to relevant projects and at right times, but the members' benefit calculations will come into play and be decisive for their further participation.

Summary – criteria for tactical planning and partnerships

As a summary of this chapter, we highlight the following requirements for HiAP regarding tactical planning and organizing in local and regional planning.

Requirements for plan content:

- The tactical plan must define relevant projects, measures, activities and changes.
- The plan must specify the background, purpose, objectives, content, organization, division of responsibilities, cost estimates, method of financing and timing of implementation for the activities in the plan.
- It must prioritize which projects, measures, activities and changes are to be carried out when (action programme).
- It must have a clear distinction between what oneself can do, what to do together with others and what only others can do.

Requirements for the HiAP planning process:

- The planning process should involve decision-making and coordination based on ethical-political discourses which are oriented towards processing conflicts of interest.
- It should have a two-dimensional view of power on the political decision-making process, that is, power decides the decision-making opportunities and the actual problems, solutions and participants.
- The process management should have the capacity to organize, prioritize, make programmes and budgets, etc.

HiAP as tactical planning must contribute to:

- Increase HiAP's capacity to make decisions and the cognitive legitimacy of HiAP.
- Reduce the scope and intensity of conflicts of interest regarding the use of resources in the public sector and between the public, private and voluntary sectors.

- Identify the key actors in the development and to strengthen weakly organized groups so that they can better look after their interests.
- Promote a flexible organization based on tactical partnerships between public, private and voluntary activities, and possibly create new organizations (projects) that can be responsible for the implementation of actions.
- Set up a binding action programme between collaborating actors.

The doings – implementation, operative planning and partnerships

Previously, we have argued that the doing can be understood as a pragmatic discourse about social actions related to cognitive and pragmatic legitimacy (see Chapter 3). This discourse is about facts and data, cost/benefit calculations and the connections between cause and effect and how this knowledge can be used to choose means to achieve given goals. The discourse is tied to the operative planning and instrumental rationality, that is planning as a activity of problem-solving, involving rational choices by self-interested individuals or homogeneous social units.

By the implementation variable, we mean the extent to which the actors and partnerships involved, alone or in collaboration with others, have the capacity and tools to follow up and implement measures and changes that can contribute to wanted and desired change. It is of course desirable that the implementation of the measures and changes are in accordance with one's own plans, but to achieve this it is required that one has power and control over the implementation process. In a power perspective, strong implementation variable means having knowledge and other resources to implement what is politically decided, but it also means being able to prevent the implementation of such decisions (Lukes, 1974). By implementing the actions, we mean the regional and local organizations' possibility to control that the implementation, is as closely as possible in accordance with visions, strategies, action programmes, etc.

The operative planning is limited both in relation to the time perspective and the theme. The purpose of operative planning is to manage production and promote efficiency so that resources are well utilized. *Operative planning* is what Alexander (2000) calls rational or, more precisely, instrumental rational planning, which is directed towards problem-solving where the actors, whether they are individuals or organizations, choose the planning solutions that give them the most benefits. Operative planning sets up specific work targets for individual activities based on institutional, strategic and tactical planning, and the preceding planning can be seen as an additional aid towards establishing the necessary legitimacy and power at the operative level. The status of the operative planning process is documented in annual budgets, development plans, development contracts etc.

Implementation in network organizations requires legitim instrumental power, therefore it is very important that the institutional, strategic and tactical planning has served as legitimizer and created a political will to support the operative planning and implementation. This support must be reflected in *operative partnerships* and concrete contractual documents. It is up to the tactical planning and the operative partnerships to formulate these documents, and to implement them. Operative planning requires commitment to the implementation of the action itself, and it therefore needs legally binding forms of cooperation, preferably in the form of detailed agreements and contracts between the parties for each individual cooperative initiative. Operative partnerships have a very high degree of formalization, mainly external given legitimacy, a limited number of members, a clear hierarchy, a well-developed specialization and have a clear focus on getting thing done.

Operative partnerships are often organized as projects and the relations between the partners are formalized with legally binding project plans based on the previous institutional, strategic and tactical planning. Active involvement from the contract partners in the collaborative planning is therefore expected, and without contract it can become impossible to keep partners accountable for action they have agreed to implement when the action is delayed, only partly implemented or there is no action at all. In principle, operative planning and partnerships do not have room for free passengers. In practice, such free passengers will normally be faced with the alternative of participating actively, withdrawing voluntarily or being excluded from the partnership.

We have experienced that strategic and tactical planning can easily gain support because, among other things, it only expresses intentions for action. Commitment to operative plans can be a problem and has often proved to be a critical point. It seems to be easy to get commitment and participation if one does not have to commit oneself to being involved in the implementation, but when implementation must be discussed, participants also drop out. To put it bluntly, one can say that some actors are involved in collaborative planning if they can set goals for others' activities. We do not think that this problem is easily solved by limiting the participation of the central actors in the implementation. We believe, and we have experience, that collaborative planning as a will formation activity over time leads to more realistic goals and a greater commitment to operative action (Amdam, 2011).

For local and regional development included HiAP, a complete will formation process must be seen as the main key to succeed. The doing needs high pragmatic legitimacy (regarded as useful), but also cognitive, normative and regulative legitimacy. At the operative level HiAP needs binding and concrete plans for each planned activity. These plans are important to coordinate the progress and to check whether each partner is implementing their part of the plans.

Summary – criteria for operative planning and partnerships

As a summary of the discussion in this chapter, we highlight the following evaluation criteria for HiAP as operative and action-oriented local and regional planning.

Requirements for HiAP document content:

- The operative actions regarding background, purpose, goal setting, management, costs and financing, implementation, quality assurance, reporting, etc. must be specified.
- There must be action contracts for the operative actions that provide for cooperation and distribution of work tasks between several autonomous actors.

Requirements for the HiAP planning process:

- The process should emphasize production and implementation based on pragmatic discourses linked to factual assessment, benefit calculations and collective priorities.
- HiAP should have a one-dimensional view of power and a focus on the output side of policy production, and the power to control that implementation is in accordance with what was intended.
- HiAP should make use of instrumental rational planning when the purpose is to programme action in a situation with agreement on goals and means.
- The planners should be programmers that can standardize, regulate, optimise, analyse, manage, etc.
- The process management should have the competence to set up binding contracts with partners, to control the partners' implementation, to sanction lack of activity, etc.

HiAP as operative planning should contribute to:

- Increase HiAP's capacity to implement decisions and the pragmatic legitimacy of HiAP.
- Reduce the scope and intensity of conflicts about facts.
- Create operative partnerships that regulate the responsibilities between the actors (action contracts).
- Carry out many individual and collective visible activities.
- Promote local control over resources and the power to improve one's own situation.

Learning, monitoring and evaluation in the continuous process of knowing

Planning and evaluation can be seen as mirror images. We agree with the World Health Organization (2001: 524) when writing that the process of evaluation is integrally related to the process of planning, and that planning, implementation and evaluation are portrayed as elements of an interactive cycle: planning leads to implementation, which leads to evaluation, which in turn can lead to further development of planning.

WHO summarizes their discussion on evaluation in five conclusions: (1) evaluation should be participatory, (2) have adequate resources, (3) examine both processes and outcomes, (4) use a mix of methodological designs and (5) evaluation expertise in complex design should be fostered (World Health Organization, 2001: 245–255).

This is in line with Habermas (1996) who writes there is no need for separate discourses for evaluation and learning, because these functions are embedded in the other discourses when they function according to the requirement of communicative rationality. This means that planning, evaluation and learning are closely linked, and that evaluation and learning must contain juridical, moral, ethical-political and pragmatic discourses and promote learning at institutional, strategic, tactical and operative level. Through reporting and evaluations, information can be obtained on both the production, the product, the efficiency and the effects of measures and changes that have been carried out. This return of knowledge can provide a basis for more active learning, better knowledge of the situation, and better knowledge of the possibilities and limitations of planning as a process. By this we mean evaluation that produces knowledge about events and actions, which can give new recognition and which can promote new practices. This can also involve assessment of deviations, error correction, quality control, etc. Through the evaluation, it is possible to check that the implementation of the measures and changes remain within the agreed resource framework, objectives, regulations and whether people are getting their needs met.

When understanding learning as a collaborative planning process, it is important to talk about learning at different levels. Bateson (1985) identifies and discusses leaning at four levels, and we have found that these levels can easily be adapted to our planning model. The four levels are:

- *Learning at 0-level* is seen as no learning at all. New situations which seem to be like earlier situations are met with the same solution (laws, legislation, manuals, standard operative procedures and other stable action models).
- *Learning at I-level* means choosing among different solutions within a set of options. In a situation with similar information as in an earlier situation, the actors can choose solutions that are appropriate to the situation.
- *Learning at II-level*. When learning reaches this level, the actor can choose among sets of options based on different values. Compared to the situation at I-level, the actors manage to evaluate and change to another set of value-based alternatives.
- *Learning at III-level* is about contextualizing learning' and is often called meta-learning and can be interpreted as learning how to learn and setting the framework for learning at different levels.

These four levels correspond to the much-used terms in learning literature as meta-learning, and triple, double and single loop learning. But instead of these learning terms, we use terms from planning literature: *learning at institutional, strategic, tactical and operative level.*

Learning at operative level indicates that rules and old praxis tell the actors what is to be adequate praxis. In given situations, one run to the standard solutions to the problems that have been used before (if your hand is in the fire, you drag the hand out off the fire). No other alternatives are regarded as possible solutions. The actors do not know any other way to act. This can be an appropriate action, but it is more likely that the action is dominated of routines, orthodoxy and can be a pervert respond to the stimuli.

Learning at tactical level is what we routinely refer to as learning in the form of generalization from basic experiences. Like you have experienced "hand in fire" and "being burned", and "I won't do it again". This learning is about evaluating action against goals, but these goals are firm and are not changed due to learning. Action and learning at this level mean that the dominating action pattern gives opportunities to discuss several possible actions, but the goal is the same.

Learning at strategic level is a kind of change of paradigm including new values, norms and ends. This learning means; "I don't generally risk getting burned, but I might do so to save someone else from a fire". In this situation, the actors not only evaluate the different alternatives to reach the goal, but they evaluate different goals. Learning at strategic level means that one will be back in learning at tactical and operative level, but now within a new kind of paradigm. Such learning happens rarely and is a kind of culture revolution that can take place both in organizations and local and regional communities. In a learning perspective, such a change is to be regarded as in depth-learning. If one wants fundamental changes, one need this *deep learning* of new values at strategic level. Persons and organizations that have learned at this level have internalized new values and adopted corresponding logical courses of action as part of their repertoire of actions. Although such deep-level learning undoubtedly takes place, it seems difficult to obtain it. For HiAP a relevant example of deep learning is getting people to take more responsibility for their own health.

To set up a system of learning that stimulates learning at all the levels, is a main issue for the institutional planning. *Learning at institutional level* appears when the referential framework evolves, and the main objectives of the organization or community are modified. Involving organizations in partnership for public health work is an example of institutional changes that create opportunities to develop new systems of learning. The institutional framework and system of learning influences the learning processes at all the other levels and must be designed very carefully to stimulate the wanted learning.

In single organizations the leaders have the overall responsibility to design adequate learning systems. In partnerships and implementation structures like HiAP, this responsibility is transformed to the leaders of the local/regional process/projects. For all these leaders the fundamental questions that must be asked continuously are what is the best way of stimulating learning at operative, tactical, strategic and institutional level. At the same time there is a need to take into consideration that all the levels of learning are interconnected within the system of learning.

However, experience shows that such systems of learning, despite good intentions, tend to include only what is measurable and what is desirable to measure. The evaluation processes therefore have a tendency of becoming very instrumental measurements of product and achievements (outputs) against the concrete operative and tactical goals (efficiency and effectiveness), and to contribute little to a learning process where the effects are compared to the strategic goals and the institutional objectives which is the basis for the actions (quality and legitimacy). See Figure 1.2.

Summary – criteria for evaluation and learning

After this, it is reasonable to point out that evaluations in connection with planning and development work is a process that contains all the same elements that planning does. In summary, we believe that the following assessment criteria should be used as a basis for evaluation and learning in HiAP.

Requirements for reporting documents:

- The reporting must include assessments of the planning and development processes, the product and the achievements and their effects measured against the content of the operative, tactical, strategic and institutional planning.
- It must contain proposals for changes in the institutional, strategic, tactical and operative planning documents.

Requirements for the evaluation process:

- The evaluation process should be a planning process that functions as a learning system that connects the actors in continuous learning processes.
- The evaluation should be a legitimation process based on juridical, moral, ethical-political and pragmatic discourses.
- It should be a process with a four-dimensional, three-dimensional, two-dimensional and one-dimensional view of power.
- It should focus on the political process's overall production, both the input side, the decision-making, the output, outcome and impact side.
- It should use adequate indicators and have a critical reflection and dialogue about what they tell.
- The evaluation should have a process/project management that stimulates learning at all learning levels.

An evaluation process must, among other things, contribute to:

- Learning at institutional, strategic, tactical and operative level.
- Obtain objective knowledge about and people's perceptions of the effects of the planning and development on the needs, demands, expectations, support and resources in society and the organization.
- Promote open democratic evaluation processes that involve both the private, public and voluntary sectors, and which through various discourses can lead to changing perceptions of reality, lead to new recognition of the desired future state, to new ways of organizing and to new measures.

Conclusion

Capacity building processes mean that people take responsibility and act collectively. To stimulate such processes, our experience shows that it is important to establish meeting places or learning arenas where the people through interaction with each other can learn through discussion and interaction, and thus also gain greater insight into the situation. If the planning and development work is carried out so that only a few people participate, the overall goal of a more capacity building and legitimizing process will be difficult to achieve, precisely because too few learn how to carry the process forward. With inspiration from Habermas (1996) and Scott (2014) on legitimating processes in political institutions, we have identified discourses, variables and tools in planning which in combination, can contribute to capacity building and increased legitimacy. We have experienced that planning processes that do not consist of all these forms of planning will fail to stimulate the various variables and to build the necessary capacity and democratic legitimacy. Furthermore, we have shown that institutional, strategic, tactical, and operative planning must combine instrumental and communicative rationality, that they can have different functions to increase the various forms of legitimacy, but only a complete planning system with all forms of planning, can give the plan and planning legitimacy and capacity. However, this process must be properly managed and monitored, which is the topic in the next chapter.

References

Alexander, E. R. 2000. Rationality revisited: Planning paradigms in a post-postmodernist perspective. *Journal of Planning Education and Research*, 19: 242–256. https://doi.org/10.1177/0739456x0001900303

Amdam, J. 1995. Mobilization, participation and partnership building in local development planning: Experience from local planning on women's conditions in six Norwegian Communes. *European Planning Studies*, 3 (3): 305–332.

Amdam, R. 1997. Empowerment planning in local communities. *International Planning Studies*, 2 (3): 329–345. http://dx.doi.org/10.1080/13563479708721688

Amdam, R. 2001. Empowering new regional political institutions - a Norwegian case. *Journal of Planning Theory & Practice*, 2 (2): 169–185. https://doi.org/10.1080/14649350120068786
Amdam, R. 2005. *Planlegging Som Handling*. Oslo: Universitetsforlaget.
Amdam, R. 2010. *Planning in Health Promotion Work: An Empowerment Model*. Abingdon, Oxon and New York: Routledge.
Amdam, R. 2011. *Planlegging og prosessleiing. Korleis lykkast i utviklingsarbeid*. Oslo: Samlaget.
Amdam, R. 2020. Planning and innovation in a collaborative framework. In: Hagen, A. & Higdem, U. (eds.) *Innovation in Public Planning. Calculate, Communicate and Innovate*. Cham, Switzerland: Palgrave Macmillan.
Amdam, R. 2021: *Kommunal handlingskapasitet. Erfaringar med ein modell for samarbeidsdriven planlegging og innovasjon*. Rapport - nr. 112/2021. Volda: Høgskulen i Volda. https://bravo.hivolda.no/hivolda-xmlui/handle/11250/2827480
Amdam, R. 2022. *Samskapt berekraft. Ei modell for samarbeidsdriven planlegging og innovasjon*. Rapport - nr. 115/2022. Volda: Høgskulen i Volda. https://bravo.hivolda.no/hivolda-xmlui/handle/11250/2991502
Bateson, G. 1985. *Steps to an Ecology of Mind*. New York: Ballantine Books.
Bennett, R. & McCoshan, A. 1993. *Enterprise and Human Resource Development. Local Capacity Building*. London: Paul Chapman Publishing.
Dryzek, J. S. 1990. *Discursive Democracy. Politics, Policy, and Political Science*. Cambridge: Cambridge University Press.
Forester, J. 1993. *Critical Theory, Public Policy and Planning Practice: Toward a Critical Pragmatism*. Albany NY: University of New York Press.
Friedmann, J. 1992. *Empowerment. The Politics of Alternative Development*. Cambridge MA and Oxford UK: Blackwell Publishers.
Giddens, A. 1984. *The Constitutions of Society: Outline of the Theory of Structuration*. Berkeley CA: University of California Press.
Habermas 1996. *Between Facts and Norms: Contributions to a Discourse Theory of Law and Democracy*. Cambridge, MA: MIT-press.
Healey, P. 1997. *Collaborative Planning. Shaping Places in Fragmented Societies*. London: Macmillan Press.
Healey, P. 1999. *Institutional Capacity-Building, Urban Planning and Urban Regenerating Projects*. Paper presented at the XII AESOP Congress. Aveiro: University of Aveiro. https://api.semanticscholar.org/CorpusID:112534533
Innes, J., Gruber, J. E., Thompson, J. & Neuman, R. 1994. *Co-Ordinating Growth and Environmental Management Through Consensus-Building*. Report to the California policy seminar. Berkeley: University of California.
Jacobsen, K. D. 1964. *Teknisk hjelp og politisk struktur*. Oslo: Universitetsforlaget.
Labonte, R. & Laverack, G. 2001a. Capacity building in health promotion, part 1: For whom? And for what purpose? *Critical Public Health*, 11 (2):111–127. https://doi.org/10.1080/09581590110039838
Labonte, R. & Laverack, G. 2001b. Capacity building in health promotion, part 2: Whose use? And with what measurement? *Critical Public Health*, 11 (2):129–138. http://dx.doi.org/10.1080/09581590110039847
Lukes, S. 1974. *Power: A Radical View*. London: Macmillan.
Lundquist, L. 1976. Några synspunkter på begreppet politisk planering. *Statsvetenskapleg Tidsskrift*, 79 (2): 121–139.
Østerud, Ø 1979. *Det planlagte samfunn. Om sentralplanleggingens fremvekst og grenser*. Oslo: Gyldendal Norsk Forlag.
Parsons, T. 1977. *Social Systems and the Evolution of Action Theory*. New York: Free Press.
Putnam, R. D. 1993. *Making Democracy Work: Civic Traditions in Modern Italy*. Princeton, NJ: Princeton University Press.

Scott, W. R. 2014. *Institutions and Organizations: Ideas, Interests, and Identities*. 4th edition. London: Sage Publications.

Stöhr, W. 1990. Synthesis, introduction and on the theory and practice of local development in Europe. In: Stöhr, W. (ed.) *Global Challenge and Local Response*. London and New York: Mansell.

Storper, M. 1997. *The Regional World. Territorial Development in a Global Economy*. New York & London: Guilford Press.

World Health Organization. 2001. *Evaluation in Health Promotion. Principles and Perspectives*. WHO regional publications European series, No. 92. Geneva: World Health Organization. https://www.who.int/publications/i/item/9789289013598

5

MANAGING AND MONITORING HiAP AS A COLLABORATIVE PLANNING PROCESS

This chapter shows that collaborative planning with institutional, strategic, tactical and operative planning can be set up to stimulate the development variables context, mobilizing, organizing and implementation, and has a potential to become a political will formation process. However, this process is not straight forward and needs both monitoring and managing to succeed. The weakest variable must be stimulated most with the right form of planning. Therefore, collaborative planning needs a meta-management of the whole process and a management that can enforce the different variables. Thus, the process manager or the process management needs to have the competence to design and monitor the process, facilitate dialogue, moderate debates, mediating conflict and execute activities. This chapter operationalizes this managing and monitoring process, and clarifies the relations between planning, democratic legitimacy and institutional capacity.

Introduction

Capacity building is an important aspect of all evaluation, but in an empowerment perspective, the capacity building process must include more than the capacity to implement defined activities and projects. This broader understanding of the capacity building process implies that improving the community's total and long-term capacity to design the process, set the political agenda, make decisions and implement planned actions is a key issue for empowerment work. If the process does not increase this capacity, the community might become less capable to solve own problems, and the community might become more dependent on external help. Lack of external support and lack of internal mobilization, organization and action can each give an incomplete process. Regardless the planners are from outside or

DOI: 10.4324/9781003451273-5

inside, we argued that monitoring the process is the most important work for the process management. This argument is in accordance with the theoretical basis for the political will formation planning model we have outlined so far in this book. All the variables in the model must be strong and active if the process shall succeed, and to stimulate the weakest variable at any time is always the most successful approach to increase capacity and legitimacy. In planning today, monitoring and learning is regarded as an integrated part of planning systems, and learning in empowerment planning and evaluation is much a similar and parallel activity. The planning and evaluation processes need to stimulate learning at institutional, strategic, tactical and operative level of the planning.

Fetterman (2005: 50) writes that the strength of empowerment evaluation is in fostering internal accountability, and empowerment evaluation is used to achieve internal goals and external requirements and outcomes, and empowerment evaluation can help organizations and communities to learn and to improve their processes and programmes. Empowerment evaluation is conducted with the purpose to improve the process, and should never be conducted for the sake of intellectual curiosity alone. The feedback loops are designed to produce information about how the process is working (or not working), and to stimulate a discussion about how to make correctives or adaptive changes.

In a comprehensive publication from WHO the principles and perspectives on evaluation in health promotion are discussed very thoroughly (World Health Organization, 2001). One of the main conclusions is that the evaluation in health promotion is an evolving field, and that one big challenge is to address the issues and problems involved in the evaluation. Increased internal and external pressure for evaluation is one of the issues. Firstly, professionals and other internal stakeholders frequently have a strong personal investment in their health promotion intervention. They often want to know whether their efforts have had a positive effect (outcome or impact evaluation) and the reasons why (process evaluation). Secondly, an increased demand for evaluation of health promotion is rooted in the pressure imposed by governmental and non-governmental funding agencies. They want evidence of effectiveness and particularly cost-related effectiveness (cost-benefit analyses), and evidence that the interventions have been, or are being, implemented as originally intended (World Health Organization, 2001: 521). Not surprisingly, the conclusion after reviewing evaluations of health promotion is a shortage of evidence on effectiveness. Data about the process and the output is normally easily accessible. To get valid data about the outcomes and impacts and then establish plausible causality between the input from the public health work and the impact on the public health work is a far more demanding and complicated. For Health in All Policies (HiAP), this shortage can be explained by several causes. Firstly, the inherent difficulty of evaluating complex interventions that involves multilevel, multi-sector and multi-strategy interventions that have a poor control over the implementation. A second cause is the lack of accepted appropriate methodologies and methods to collect evidence of effectiveness, quality and legitimacy.

Nicola and Hatcher (2000) discuss a framework and guidance on building effective public health constituencies to achieve community health improvement and compare different planning approaches from a leadership perspective. They write that knowing the community is essential because social programme tends to fail due to lack of appropriate management and an oversimplified view of essential motivation. They argue that knowing the community and its citizens is more than epidemiological assessment, and if public health leaders view networking as an ongoing and essential activity in the agency's operations, community mobilization can be productive and require minimal efforts. Likewise, Wilson (2004: 409) argues that national health programmes need to be structured in a way that balances the advantages of regional approaches to public health challenges with the benefits of a coordinated central response, and the policymakers need to address the unique challenges of the public health governance.

Laverack and Labonte (2000: 257) argue that to ensure community capacity building, and community empowerment, it is best to see the process as an integrated two parallel structure with a programme track and an empowerment track, which are linked during the progressive stages of the programme implementation process:

- Overall programme design,
- objective setting,
- strategy selection,
- strategy implementation,
- and programme evaluation.

Their intention is to provide us with a planning framework for incorporating community empowerment into top-down health promotion programme. We find their framework a good description of some of the challenges of combining the top-down and bottom-up implementation, but their framework seems to build on a linear form of planning without discussing all the limitations such a linear process has when used on a continuous process like public health work. A more circular model is provided by Tones (1974) and Tones and Green (2004). They describe a systems checklist for health promotion. The model combines an education and cognitive affective behavioural change process, with an environment and supportive policy process. The model incorporates a lot of variables that we find relevant for a planning process, but the model may be too complex when used as approach to HiAP.

Network organizations in need of process monitoring and management

Government and governance can both be characterized by its ability to make decisions and its capacity to enforce them. The main difference between them is that organizations within government rest on resources under the authority and sanctions of the government. Governance is a network structure which cannot be externally imposed but is the outcome of the interaction of influencing actors in a multi-actor process. Stoker (2004: 27) talks about the *network community governance* as an emerging new form of management. He concludes his discussion that network community governance marks a break from Traditional Public Administration and New Public Management in its vision of the role of local government and its understanding of the context for governing and the core process of governance. In the network community governance, the overarching goal is greater effectivity in tackling the problems that public sector most care about. He maintains that no sector has the monopoly on public sector ethos, that relationships are maintained through shared values, and that network governance is seemingly a return to a more value-based governance and a restoration of core public sector values such as separated powers, democracy, transparency, accountability, equity and effectiveness.

The term *network organizations* can be used as a collective term for collaboration and partnership in local and regional planning and development, which covers multi-levels and multi-sectors cooperations, that is governing bodies that are comprised of actors from the vertical and the horizontal power structures. Common to all of them is the fact that the collaborating organizations can have a large degree of independence, and that they can disappear from the network, either of their own free will or because the partners choose to exclude them. Network organizations are normally loosely coupled organizations, and therefore obtain the power and legitimacy the different collaborating organizations want to give them, and the power the context can accept (Strand, 2001). Networks are political arenas in the intersection between vertical and horizontal power, and between functional and territorial logic, but not in such a way that one dominates the other. If the power imbalance becomes a pattern, the losing actors in the network organizations will respond by withdrawing, and the multi-dimensional policy will fall apart.

Network organizations operate initially in environments which are typical for trust-based transactions, that is control mechanism is characterized by low levels of task programmability and low levels of output measurability. The contracts are broad frameworks, which tend to develop further in detail over time. The context is complex and changing, and the performance has low repetitiveness. The initial selection of partners is based on perceptions of trust which arise through friendship, reputation and formal contractual relationship. The contracts tend to grow out of the need for formalization of the cooperations. However, problems can arise when the participating organizations, which are most familiar with market-based (private sector) and bureaucratic-based (public sector) transaction control mechanism, shall form powerful network organizations based on trust. These problems have arisen with the New Public Management reforms because these reforms seem to have transformed public sector away from trust-based relationships in Traditional Public Administration to more *mistrust-based* transactions in New Public Management.

Network organizations are based on interdependency, trust and mutual interest of achieving outcome they cannot create alone. Participating in network organizations is normally formalized through agreements and transaction control mechanisms between the participants. In theory the control mechanism in network organizations can be based on market, bureaucracy or trust (Langfield-Smith & Smith, 2003: 286). But accountability deficit does often become a problem, because actors in network organizations have a significant degree of autonomy and are driven by self-interest of their members rather than a wider concern with the public interest or particularly those excluded from the network (Stoker, 1998: 24).

For governance the ultimate partnership activity is to form self-governing network (Stoker, 1998: 23). Here, we like to highlight Ansell and Gash's (2007) meta-analysis of 137 theoretical and empirical case studies on governance network where they identified critical factors, both structural and relational, which are of great importance for the development of collaboration between different organizations. At the same time, they write that the analysis must not be understood as complete or final, but as a basis for empirical testing and theory development. They argue that the analysis can function as a framework for further research with the aim of identifying key challenges and causal connections. They compile their findings into a model that has five main characteristics (Ansell & Gash, 2007):

1 A collaborative process requires an institutional design with frameworks for the process with requirements for openness and broad participation, for forums and other meeting places, and with clear rules of the game and mandate, etc. The design must take care of and promote the acceptance and legitimacy of the process.
2 A starting situation that may be characterized by asymmetric power, knowledge and resources, by relationships that inhibit and promote participation, and a history of a lot of cooperations or conflicts. All these factors affect the collaborative process.
3 The collaborative process is referred to as an interactive and circular learning process where face-to-face dialogue is necessary but not sufficient to promote trust and respect between the actors. Increased trust will, in turn, influence adherence to and ownership of the process, the recognition of mutual dependence and the will to change.
4 Governance must of course produce results in both the short and long term, and both concrete measurable results and have a positive impact on the central values in society and on the collaborative process's capacity for action and legitimacy.
5 Furthermore, governance requires a facilitating leadership that places emphasis on maintaining clear rules of the game, building trust, facilitating dialogue and exploring mutual gains. Where incentives to participate are weak, where power and resources are asymmetrically distributed and where previous contradictions are high, leadership becomes even more important.

We find their framework and critical factors very relevant for governance processes and for HiAP as radical New Public Governance, and for monitoring and managing the will formation planning process. We regard the communicative process as the most critical factor in governance and HiAP, and according to radical New Public Governance one expects that the actors are influenced in dialogue and that they can learn, further that they can act reasonably towards others by acting altruistic more than egoistic. The interests of the society are agreed upon in broad democratic processes that include both evidence-based and experience-based knowledge, and the inhabitants are all perceived as citizens who can participate actively in both problem definition and problem-solving. The purpose of participation is to involve the people in competence building so that they can handle their own and society's problems to a greater extent, and the participation shall contribute to learning and capacity building both on a collective and individual level in network organizations and partnerships. See Chapter 2.

In communicative processes, actors can submit their understanding of the problem and how the problem influence them, but they must also listen to others telling their versions of the same. Based on our action research we have learned that critical factors in collaborative processes are, that the actors recognize that they are mutually dependent on each other, that they see themselves as equals, practice have face-to-face dialogue, share mutual understanding and have trust in each other. The partnerships must be subject to public transparency, accountability and democratic control, and must of course perform output and outcome (Amdam, 2011). See Figure 5.1.

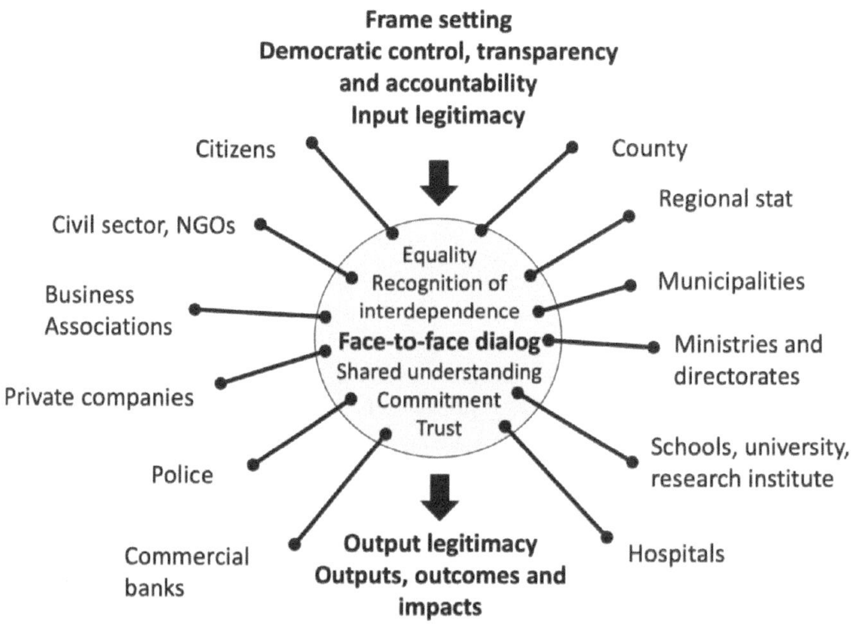

FIGURE 5.1 Critical factors in collaborative processes and partnerships

A main challenge in governance is getting the various actors to individually carry out their part of the problem-solving that they jointly have come up with. To some extent, the accountability and responsibility can be regulated through agreements, but often planned actions can stop because the actors end up in a cross-pressure between accountability to the network and to their own organization and/or profession (Synnevåg, Amdam & Fosse, 2018). Structural forces will always be a part of planning processes, but a skilled planner as process-leader must be able to contribute to a situation in which self-interests are united to promote common interests. In this perspective governance is not a fixed structure, but an institutional capacity building process (Healey, 1999, 2005). Governance, partnership, networks and coalitions must be constructed and managed (Amin & Thrift, 1994).

Metagovernance and different roles of process management

In all multi-actor system, there will be a need for someone in charge, someone who is able to conduct metagovernance (Sørensen & Torfing, 2009, 2017). According to Torfing, Sørensen and Røiseland (2016: 20), this means defining, supporting, designing and intervening in collaborative networks while simultaneously respecting their capacity for self-regulation. Thus, in local and regional planning there is a need for governing the governance and to set the frames for collaborative processes, while taking account of the context by reinforcing, counteracting and possibly changing the institutional structural forces in society. This means that politicians must have the power to create, close, change and control the collaborative networks that are part of the local and regional planning.

The structural forces are a constant threat to the existence of collaborative partnerships. Selznick (1957: 55–56) highlights four central tasks leaders are set to perform when consideration is given to the organization's character or institutional features: (1) To defend institutional integrity and prevent the organization from external pressure, (2) to define institutional goals, (3) to institutionalize purposes in administrative management, organizational design, delegation, etc. and (4) to master internal conflicts. He emphasizes that over time, organizations develop institutional features with their own values, norms, processes and cultures. It is therefore important to have institutional leadership that provides direction, positions and motivates. We regard this statement valid for organizations as well as network organizations.

But collaborative processes are often marked by an imbalance of power between the actors because they have different interests, different resources to argue for their opinions, and different capacities to participate in the implementation. It is of course a requirement of the processes that one should try to equalize such inequality, but in situations with citizens with low argumentative power and low capacity for action, it will often require a high degree of intervention and mobilization to achieve capacity building among all citizens. Therefore, the process managers in such processes must also be aware of their own role, and gradually withdraw so that the citizen can experience mastery and capacity building. Only in this way equality and a balance of power can be established. Or as Bryson, Crosby and Bloomberg (2014: 448) write: "In the new approach, government agencies can be conveners, catalysts, and collaborators – sometimes steering, sometimes rowing, sometimes partnering, and sometimes staying out of the way."

Agger and Sørensen (2018) have studied how frontline planners manage collaborative innovation processes, and through a synthesis of collaborative planning theory, and theories of network governance and public innovation, they have identified several tensions, and four coping strategies planners use in different situations: *pilot*, *whip*, *culture-maker* and *communicator*. Ansell and Gash (2012) identify three coping strategies: stewards, mediators and catalysts. Similarly, Torfing (2016) writes that the actors in collaborative innovation act as *conveners*, *facilitators* and *catalysts*, but he also writes that collaborative innovation requires a transformative and distributed leadership.

How planners act can be described in many ways, and the planning theorist John Forester has helped us to understand the role as planners working in government agencies. He has explicitly taken pragmatism into planning by introducing the term "critical pragmatism". Thus, Forester (2012) combines a pragmatic approach with Jürgen Habermas's communicative theory on social actions in public sphere contexts, and Forester has identified planners' pragmatic approach to planning as they *facilitate dialogues*, *moderate debates* and *mediate conflicts* in different contexts. In addition to the three roles that Forester (2012) writes about, we add and highlight the important role the planner has as a framework setter and interpreter of the context and essential laws and rules, guidelines, plans and decisions. These roles involve understanding and interpreting the institutional framework that planning must take as a starting point, but the role can also be to challenge and change structural forces in the established framework.

Into this process, all the actors will bring with them all their experiences from previous actions, and their knowledge, skills, values and ability to act. This means that all the participants will use their wisdom or competence in institutional planning and management. In practice, the participants meet in discussions where some may have a lot of competence and others less, and together they can challenge and complement each other so that both individual and collective competence can increase and contribute to higher democratic legitimacy and institutional capacity. See Chapter 4.

Managing and monitoring a collaborative planning process

What planning, management and leadership have in common is that they involve exercising political power, and in democratic countries this exercise of power must have democratic legitimacy. In political processes, institutional action capacity is understood as the power to translate words and thoughts into action. According to

Lukes (1974), power in political processes can be divided into several dimensions (see Chapter 1), which we interpret like this:

- The four-dimensional power expresses the institutional planning's capacity to handle external challenges and to set frames and design the planning process, including progress, content and participants.
- The three-dimensional power expresses the strategic planning's capacity to mobilize and to set the political agenda.
- The two-dimensional power expresses the tactical planning's capacity to organize resources and make binding decisions.
- The one-dimensional power expresses the operative planning's capacity to implement decisions.

Common to all four dimensions is that power will also trigger counter-power, and that actors can prevent problems from being on the agenda, that decisions are made, that actions are taken and that the direction is challenged. Thus, the power and capacity to act, are dependent of being accepted and legitimized. And according to Scott (2002, 2014) different pillars and mechanisms in an organization's contexts maintain an institution's legitimacy. We interpret his regulative, normative and cognitive mechanisms to belong to the public sphere and the institutional context, and pragmatic legitimacy to belong to an instrumental technical context with cost-benefit calculations. When adapted to our communicative planning approach the different forms of legitimacy can be expressed like this:

- Institutional planning maintains the regulative legitimacy through delivering processes and impacts in accordance with laws, rules, regulations, plans and overall societal values (democratic legitimacy).
- Strategic planning maintains the normative legitimacy through delivering processes and outcomes that satisfies the needs (quality).
- Tactical planning maintains the cognitive legitimacy through delivering processes and outcomes that fulfil quantified goals (effectiveness).
- Operative planning maintains the pragmatic legitimacy through delivering processes and outputs that are cost-benefit effective (efficiency)

Based on research into collaborative processes and collaborative planning, management and leadership, we have put together a model with the different forms of legitimacy and action capacity seen in relation to different forms of planning (Amdam, 2022, 2023). See Table 5.1. We present the connection between the various forms of legitimacy, capacity and planning as a staircase. We call the model *the planning staircase*, but the model is relevant for both management and leadership. In the model, certain forms of legitimacy and power are related to the various forms of planning, and in the model, these are marked *as dark grey* and form the

TABLE 5.1 Major relations between planning, capacity and legitimacy – the planning staircase

Forms of legitimacy	**Regulative legitimacy**	**Normative legitimacy**	**Cognitive legitimacy**	**Pragmatic legitimacy**
Forms of action capacity	Process and results are in accordance with laws, etc.	Process and outcomes satisfy important needs	Process and outcomes fulfil quantified goals	Process and outputs are useful
Power to handle external challenges and to set frames and design the planning process	*Institutional planning* *To know WHY* *Metagovernance*			
Power to mobilize people and to set the political agenda		*Strategic planning* *To know WHAT* *Facilitate dialogs*		
Power to organize resources and make binding decisions			*Tactical planning* *To know HOW* *Moderate debates*	
Power to implement decisions				*Operative planning* *DOING* *Mediate conflicts*

steps in the staircase. It is important that all steps in the staircase are solid so that the planning, management and leadership achieve a strong capacity for action and a high degree of legitimacy. But this does not mean that the other forms of planning, management and leadership are not important (non-text areas in the model). All the 16 areas count when the exercise of power is to be legitimized, but the main weight of the planning must be put into making the stairs and steps as solid as possible.

Here it must be pointed out that the regulative legitimacy of formally adopted laws, regulations, cooperation agreements, etc. has come about through its own legitimation processes where both pragmatic, cognitive, normative and regulative conflicts have been resolved and the solutions are built into the regulative text. The text of laws, regulations, etc. thus provide guidance on how both regulative, normative, cognitive and pragmatic conflicts should be handled in practice.

In Amdam (2022) we document that the systematic use of this model as a tool can increase the legitimacy and action capacity of collaboration. Our experience shows that the process cannot be linear, but that process manager must continuously check whether the stair and the steps are strong enough by moving up and down the staircase to strengthen the various steps. The process managers must therefore be busy with institutional, strategic, tactical and operative planning at the same time to ensure sufficient legitimacy and capacity for action for the process and the results. The role as process manager thus becomes interpreting laws, regulations and other guidelines, facilitating dialogues, moderating debates and mediating conflicts more or less simultaneously. Our experience suggests that if planning, management and leadership are to give plans and decisions a high degree of legitimacy and capacity, all these forms of planning must be fulfilled, and that all involved participate in the process with their expertise.

Institutional planning and metagovernance

We regard institutional planning as the process of knowing why and as a juridical discourse about social values related to pragmatic and normative legitimacy with strong regulative implications. The main purpose of institutional planning is to maintain and increase the regulative legitimacy and the power to design the planning process. Learning at institutional level can be called metalearning or learning how to learn and is expressed with changed frame setting and process design. The management role is what is called metagovernance with the main purpose to scan the process, to determine which capacity and legitimacy are the weakest, and to choose the right form of planning to increase them. See Table 5.1.

Through institutional planning the social power from the previous moral, political-ethical and pragmatic discourses is transformed into laws and regulations and into administrative power as frames for the strategic, tactical and operative planning. Institutional planning contains moral and social obligations that describe what is appropriate behaviour and the right thing to do which become established and internalized over time. The institutional planning can tell what kind of social values such as democracy, justice, equality and resilience should be important, further applicable laws and regulations, requirements for achieving targets and reporting results, awarding of permits, etc.

From our experiences these are some of the challenges for the metagovernance to handle:

- The balance between top-down and bottom-up politics.
- The interaction between national programmes and local processes.
- Using projects to stimulate continuous processes.

Institutional planning is a systematic process for developing a frame of reference for future decisions and actions by a local and region community. If we compare our understanding of this process with Laverack and Labonte (2000:

258) model of community capacity building, the term institutional planning covers what they call overall programme design with the elements programme size, time frame, role of outside agent and participation especially from marginalized populations. In Selznick's (1957: 55–56) terms managing institutional planning is to defend institutional integrity and prevent the organization from external pressure. Thus, the institutional planning should have institutional capacity building and enforcing the local power structure as its superior objective. This means a struggle where the alliance between the civil society and the elected representatives fight to make the communicative rationality superior to the instrumental rationality in their communities. The process needs to involve actors from public, private and voluntary sectors and from local, regional and national level. Local and regional communities can influence their own development and stand up as political institutions with legitimacy and power, if they are able to create a policy legitimating process. Hence, the locally based cross-sector power can become a counter force and challenge the established vertical power structure in government.

Essentially the institutional planning concerns the relations between the community and the structural powers in the context that create both opportunities and obstacles for the local and regional communities as political actors. In concrete terms, that means that the building up of an institutional capacity in a local or region community takes place in interaction with the surroundings. Therefore, the planning must attempt to bring to light structural forces in the context and to determine to what extent they represent opportunities or threats for the community.

Institutional planning at regional and local level focuses on knowing why to change something and must strengthen the regulative legitimacy and the capacity to act to design the process and to interpret and set framework and require someone to take responsibility for managing the process. In many contexts, local and regional development work is included in national and international programmes, and then the programme itself will form a framework for how the development work can be carried out. Furthermore, the local and regional actors' own plans and guidelines will also act as frameworks for the development work.

The institutional public health planning must contribute to increasing regulatory legitimacy and increase the capacity to convert HiAP into a local mandate for the development process. Public health programmes are often initiated nationally or internationally and implemented in local communities. A good balance between top-down policy and bottom-up policy is needed if a community shall avoid becoming dependent on external institutions to solve their problems. For these programmes the concept of *implementation chains* captures the complex meeting between top-down and bottom-up policies between the formal public levels and between the public, private and voluntary sectors. Partnerships in such chains are established between formally independent actors who cooperate because they are mutually dependent on each other to satisfy needs and promote overall societal goals (Gjertsen & Halkier, 2004). In public health work, one can talk about a public health chain from state level via county and municipalities to local communities and, finally, to individuals. A chain that involves both the public, private, voluntary and elected sectors at all levels of governing. HiAP is an example of such multi-stakeholder collaboration involving supranational, national, regional and local units organized as partnerships that are part of an implementation chain that need to constantly seek legitimacy and capacity, both from the partners and from other relevant actors. So instead of looking at implementation chains as permanent structures, HiAP should function as an institution-building process with both institutional, strategic, tactical and operative planning and partnerships. The operative planning and partnerships at one level will thus be a starting point and a frame for the institutional planning at partnerships at the level below. In this way, planning at one level can support the planning at a lower level with much needed resources, power, acceptance and legitimacy through institutional partnership agreements. Or, to put it another way, on operative action in a project at one level can give birth to institutional planning and a new project at a lower level, see Figure 5.2.

We usually organize the planning and development effort in regional and local communities as a project with a steering group as the coordinating body, and we

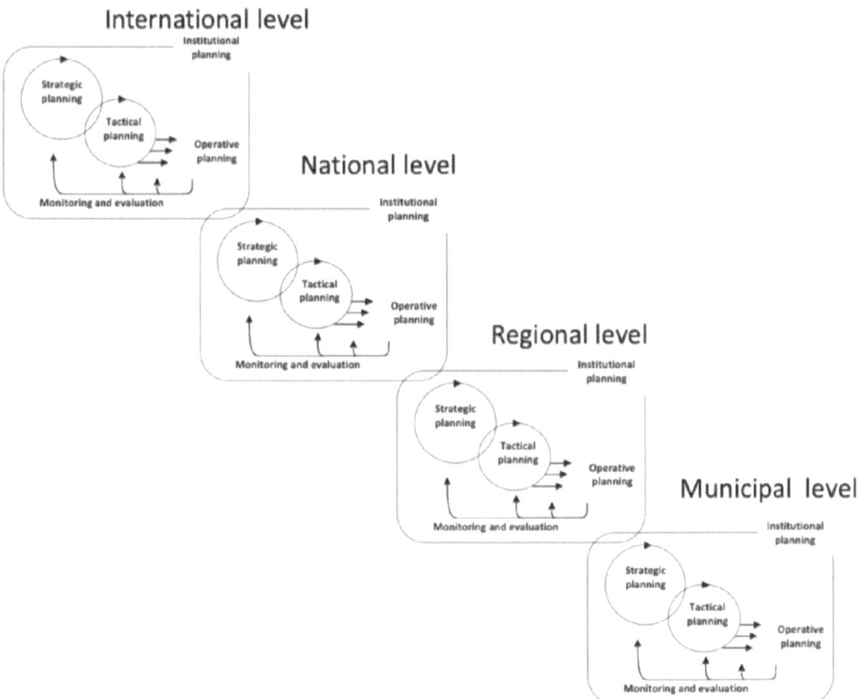

FIGURE 5.2 National development programmes as implementation chains

Source: Amdam (2010: 66).

often set up a team for teaching, supervising and evaluation. The main purpose for the project is to stimulate mobilizing, organizing, implementing and learning processes in the community, and to produce plan documents with institutional, strategical, tactical, operative and evaluating content. The local process or project will usually not to give the process and plan sufficient legitimacy and capacity. Local and regional planning exist in the interface between actors from both the vertical and horizontal power structure, and the collaborating actors are in the special situation of needing approval and legitimacy from both structures. That is, from the governing levels; municipality, county and state, and from the governing systems; voluntary, private and public sectors including democratically elected representatives. In practical planning this implies that, the planning process must incorporate actors from both the horizontal and vertical structure, and that the planning documents must be formally accepted in the appropriate organizations that belong to the two structures.

For those who build up network organizations, there is therefore a lot of power in being able to select the member organizations. At the same time, it is also the case that the work of network organizations depends on whether the member organization is equipped with strong or weak mandates. Such circumstances must be clarified in contractual cooperation at an institutional level through institutional planning and reflected in agreements/contracts that can be called institutional partnerships. Such partnerships must be understood as frameworks for relatively long-term collaboration between several organizations that see the value in collaborating on more than individual matters. Partnership agreements therefore apply to network organizations where the actors must be equal and must recognize that they are mutually dependent on each other to solve problems and satisfy needs in society. Network organizations need to justify themselves and win the trust and acceptance of both subordinates and superiors, and thus also depend on a well-functioning and complete capacity building and legitimizing process (Bache & Olsson, 2001). Purely logically, network organizations will therefore receive the acceptance and legitimacy that the member organizations give them, and the acceptance and legitimacy that the network organizations themselves manage to build up.

It is important to emphasise that regional and local planning and development work can be intensified by way of a project, but that it is none the less a continuous process. Organizing development work as a project can be a useful method of approach when an all-out effort is required for a limited period in a limited area. A well-established project presupposes that the members of the steering group have arrived at a reasonable degree of agreement about aims and means, and not least about the limits of and the mandate for the project. If one chooses to organize the intervention as a project, as often done, the superior perspective for the project should be how the project for a limited time, can influence the continuous process which development really is. One of the most severe mistakes that can be done, is to see the intervention and the project as a process for making planning documents. When this mistake is done, the process is often limited to the strategic and tactical planning and not to stimulating the mobilizing, organizing, implementing and learning variables. The will formation process becomes incomplete.

These are questions about institutional planning that process manager and the partners must ask themselves consciously to manage the HiAP process/project:

- How well is the question why HiAP addressed and accepted in the local/regional community?
- What have you as a partner or manager done to stimulate the regulative legitimacy and power to design the process of the public health work in your organization and your community/district/county?
- What are the most important outcomes and the most significant impacts on public health situation from the public health work?
- How strong is the regulative legitimacy and the capacity to design the process/project in your organization and your community/district/county?
- What is your process/project planning to do to stimulate the legitimacy and capacity?
- How does the planner/process manager execute the role as *frame setter* in your process/project?
- What are the biggest challenges for your process/project now?

Strategic planning and facilitating dialogs

We regard strategic planning as the process of knowing what and as a moral discourse about theories of reality related to normative and regulative legitimacy. The main purpose is to sustain and increase the normative legitimacy and the power to influence the political agenda. See Table 5.1. Strategic planning is about what matters for the citizens and for the community and are often expressed with visions and strategies for handling the most important challenges. Learning at strategic level is a kind of change of paradigm including new values, norms and ends. At this level the actors do not only evaluate the different alternatives to reach the goal, but they evaluate different gaols.

Planning and learning at strategic level means a process of making sense and involves a moral dimension (Etzioni, 1988, 1993), and can only be achieved through interaction and democratic discourses (Forester, 1993). This implies establishing a process of legitimating strategic policies; a process based on undistorted discourses seeking equality of power and demand for stating reasons in open public meetings. This process must be democratically inclusive and concerned with consensus building. This kind of management by arguments (Healey, 1997) is important for mutual learning, but agreements on strategies are likely to be incomplete and unstable when it comes to practice, especially if they are not founded in a collective moral.

The strategic planning concerns the interpretation, discussion and recognition of important development features and challenges, the perspective is long-term, and the content should ideally be able to remain unchanged for some time. In other words, to agree on a political agenda and build up a collective capacity for action. This is at the core of mobilizing and strategic planning. The political agenda is never stabile, and there is an enduring power battle about being high up on the agenda.

Comparing this process with Laverack and Labonte (2000: 258) model of community capacity building, the term strategic planning covers what they call objective setting and where the top-down programme objectives meet the community empowerment objectives. In Selznick's (1957: 55–56) terms managing strategic planning is to define institutional goals.

From our experiences managing institutional planning is facing several challenges (Amdam, 2011):

- The balance between evidence knowledge and local knowledge.
- Communicative processes shall generate political will.
- Direct democracy in competition to indirect democracy.
- Getting from mobilization to implementation.

Strategic planning is about knowing what, that is, developing knowledge about what kind of relevant knowledge one should emphasize to understand the situation one is in and what one should do. This knowledge should develop in broad communicative processes where both evidence-based and experience-based knowledge are mixed. Strategic plans therefore contain a specification of how one wants the situation to be, a compilation of how one experiences the situation, and what development features and challenges must be tackled to achieve the desired situation. Strategic planning is a mobilizing process to get people involved in communicative discourses about the situation for the local and regional community now and in the future, and on formulating a vision of the desired future. The process should function as a broad learning process encouraging personal growth in the entire population of the local and regional community. In this way, a local social power can be created which can further be transformed into a political power through organizing and implementing.

Strategic planning refers to fundamental questions such as what is typical for the situation with its development characteristics and challenges, what sort of future do one want, where should one start and how can one make changes to move from the present situation in the direction of a more ideal situation. Strategic planning is therefore suitable for capturing the major lines of development and for focusing on the biggest challenges. Although the environment may be changing, the main challenges may still be reasonably stable over time. Strategic planning can therefore be carried out locally and regionally as a peak effort for a limited period in, for example, a four-year cycle, and can be embodied in a guiding planning document that contains the area of effort and development pattern. Our experience suggests that if the strategic planning is to function as such a guideline for development, the content of the strategic planning must be both known and recognized. Broad participation in mobilizing processes around strategic planning seems to be able to contribute to strengthening the plan as a widely accepted target document. But, where the recognition of the development trend and the challenges is weak and scattered, it can take a long time to mobilize people and reach a commune understanding of the situation.

In public health the intervention will always be an arena where the bottom-up policymaking meets the top-down policymaking, or where the community knowledge meets the evidence-based knowledge in setting up national development programmes. Evidence-based knowledge has much to offer the development programmes; in essence they offer programme strategies or interventions that have worked in other similar communities. However, evidence-based knowledge can and shall not be blindly adopted and expected to work in new communities. If combined with the community knowledge, they should be considered as useful ideas and models potentially adaptable to the local context. Many communities have suffered when the interventions have been out of-touch with the local environment, culture, and conditions (Fetterman, 2005: 48). Local and regional community members have invaluable knowledge and information about their community. Respecting the community knowledge is important in HiAP. The local knowledge, if mobilized, can be an extraordinary catalyst for change.

Strategic public health planning must contribute to high normative legitimacy and capacity to put HiAP on the national and local political agenda and gain commitment to HiAP from actors outside the health sector. Strategic planning with the focuses on facilitating dialogues with broad participation and fostering a common understanding of what to do can be the tool to increase the normative legitimacy of HiAP, the commitment to HiAP and to put HiAP on the political agenda. In this planning, communicative rationality is important to practise, and in the communicative processes the role of the process manager is to be a facilitator of dialogues in open forums. However, in political processes there will be a constant struggle about the political agenda, and mobilizing for HiAP must therefore be a continuous process. The content of the strategic planning should reflect the level of recognition the participants are at. Broad participation is reported as important tools in the problem assessment and interpretation, and a main goal for the strategic planning is to put health promotion on the political agenda and to include health promotion activities in the planning documents.

Our experience is that such broad public meetings can have a very mobilizing and stimulating effect on the people to make an effort for the community. Collective perceptions of both the past and future situation, willingness to change and expectations that something will happen can be created. But we register big differences in how realistic these perceptions are. In several villages, municipalities, counties and regions in which we have worked, and where mobilization for the community has been weak, the first public meeting has shown that the people overestimate their own control over the situation they are in, and that they easily get very unrealistic perceptions about what they can achieve in a short time and with limited resources. In other contexts, we find that the participants have a sober perception of their own limitations and opportunities. This means that they have come relatively far in a learning process where they have drawn knowledge and recognition from their own actions. In such contexts, the public meeting becomes just one of many learning arenas in a continuous mobilization process.

One of the bottlenecks that we have registered many times is that this collective will is not translated into organizational power to implement actions. Partly because existing organizations are unable to do anything with the strategic proposals. Partly because new organizations, or collaborations between organizations, are not being established. In all cases, we experience the time factor as very important. Seen in relation to the expectations of the participants in the mobilization process, it often takes far too long in the public sector from the discussion at the public meeting for actions to show up in practice. In many cases, actions do not occur at all within what the people perceive as a reasonable time. This has a frustrating effect on the participants and leads to a form of negative learning that may make it even more difficult to mobilize later.

I addition, there is criticism from the elected and administrative leaders in the local and regional communities that the public meetings that discuss strategic issues are pure wishful thinking, and do not appear to be responsible governing bodies. It has proven to be a consistent problem that many of the elected representatives do not engage in the public meeting. There seems to be a form of conflict between the direct and the representative democracy that comes to light in that the elected representatives refuse to participate in such direct democracy as the open public meeting represents.

To increase the strategic planning's normative legitimacy and power to influence the political agenda, planners need to have the skills to facilitate broad and inclusive dialogs, and these are monitoring and self-evaluation questions that partners and manager of HiAP process/projects must ask themselves continuously about the strategic planning:

- How well is the question what matters for a successful HiAP addressed and answered in the local/regional community?
- What have you as a partner or manager of HiAP process/project done to increase normative legitimacy and put public health on the political agenda in your organization and your community/district/county?
- How accepted is HiAP as an overall goal and guideline for more detailed planning in your organization and your local or regional community now?

- What is your process/project planning to do to mobilize people to participate in the realization of HiAP?
- How do the planner/process manager execute the role as *facilitator of dialogs* in the process/project?

Tactical planning and moderating debates

We regard tactical planning as the process of knowing how and as an ethical-political discourses about political decided detailed plan for action related to regulative and cognitive legitimacy. Tactical planning has the main purpose to maintain and increase the cognitive legitimacy and the power to make binding decisions. See Table 5.1. Making tactical decisions concern the conflicts of interest that often relate to the utilization of resources. These conflicts are right at the core of the tactical planning whose aim is to obtain and deploy resources among responsible actors. Cognitive legitimacy is supported by established cultures and therefore represents a form of orthodoxy with a common logic of action. Hence, in a situation with similar information as in an earlier situation, the actors can prefer well-known solutions. Learning at tactical level often means choosing among different solutions within a set of options which expresses the inherent orthodoxy.

If we compare this understanding of tactical planning with Laverack and Labonte (2000) model of community capacity building, the term tactical planning includes what they call strategy selection included resource mobilization, links with others and organizational structures. In Selznick's (1957: 55–56) terms tactical planning is to institutionalize the organization's purposes in administrative management, organizational design, delegation, etc. In a power perspective this involves having the authority to make decisions, or to prevent decisions being taken.

Organizing and coordination are central themes in tactical planning, because the implementation of many concrete measures normally must be carried out by the collaborating organizations in partnerships. In this way, organizing becomes a critical tool in taking the step from mobilization to implementation. From our experiences managing tactical planning is facing several challenges (Amdam, 2011):

- Lack of responsibility and accountability.
- Resistance from the orthodoxies.
- A battlefield between norms and benefits.

Tactical planning is about knowing how to proceed to change what one wants and must strengthen the cognitive legitimacy and capacity to make decisions about coordination of the use of resources. The tactical planning is holistic in the sense that it has the intention in all circumstances to coordinate the activities of the planning unit. The tactical planning concerns the acquisition, development and organization of the resources. The overall prerequisite for planning at this level thus becomes to set up an action programme which distributes responsibility for the implementation, and to develop partnerships, networks and other forms of cooperation between the actors. To take responsibility is a prerequisite for this planning, but often there is a lack of delivered responsibility in the communities. We have learned that in tactical planning it is important to distinguish between the measures and changes that one can implement oneself, in collaboration with others and those that only others can implement. Therefore, tactical planning is about setting up short-term action programmes, organize cross-sectoral working groups, involving private and voluntary sectors in community development projects, etc.

However, these programmes of action can only consider how to use the organization's own resources such as money and labour, but programmes of action can stimulate producing of realistic ideas about just what the local and regional organizations are in a position to achieve, alone and in tactical partnerships. We have learned that in partnerships lack of responsibility and accountability is a main challenge in local and regional action programmes and that tactical partnerships have problem with keeping the partners accountable for the outcome, and lack of outcome. Therefore, it is very important when local and regional actions programmes are set up, that each collaborating organization takes responsibility for its part of the actions in the programme, and gets that part prioritized in their own organizations and action programmes.

In public health planning there are several organizations with separate fields of operation, and in many cases the actors must cooperate if they are to succeed in their struggle for an intended development. The establishment of these tactical partnerships requires the actors share a common understanding of the present and the future. This involves transforming social power into political power by having the people commit themselves to existing and new organizations which can accomplish through action the wanted operations and changes. The latter means that tactical planning with proposals to use resources and introduce ways of acting contrary to the way things have been before, will challenge what can be called the culture and orthodoxy in the organizations and communities. Such cultures can often take a long time to change, and therefore it is important that tactical plans are backed with high regulatory and normative legitimacy so that it is possible for a democratic majority to rule over a minority in prioritizing the recourses. Thus, the transformation of traditional public health policy to HiAP implies the capacity to challenge the orthodoxy both within the government and among people, and high cognitive legitimacy expresses the extent to which the HiAP approach is understood and accepted. Tactical public health planning must contribute to high cognitive legitimacy of public health work and to the power to make binding decisions.

We have experienced that tactical planning often becomes a battlefield between extreme argument based on the wishes from the strategic planning and extreme argument saying that almost all new actions are unrealistic based on the operative planning and the capacity to implement. This tactical debate is between actors fronting visions and actors being realistic and need to be moderated to reach a consensus. The outcome of the battle is normally compromises linked together in an incremental process where only small changes of direction can be obtained. However, small changes in right direction can over time sum up to big changes. Thus, in addition to plan for the big changes, is it important to have a clear focus on the small changes and create a lasting platform for common actions.

Conflicts about organizing and the use of resources can sometimes be solved through exercising instrumental top-down power alone, but more often moderated debates are necessary to create as large a degree of agreements as possible. In tactical planning, it often becomes very clear that the communicative and instrumental logics meet; normative and altruistic thinking meets pragmatic and individual utility thinking. The process manager's role will therefore be to moderate debates in arenas with affected actors. In this process, resistance to changed resource allocation and new actions may be more or less significant, and extreme standpoints need to be moderated if common and supported action programmes and actions are to be implemented.

These are self-evaluation questions that partners and manager of HiAP process/projects must ask themselves continuously about tactical planning:

- How well is the question how to proceed for a successful HiAP addressed and answered in the local/regional community?
- What have you as a partner or manager of HiAP process/project done to increase cognitive legitimacy and the capacity to get public health activity decided and organized in your organization and your community/district/county?
- How deeply rooted is public health work in action plans, budgets and daily work in your organization and with your partners in the community/district/county now?
- What is your process/project planning to do to get new public health activities decided and organized?
- How do the planner/process manager execute the role as *moderator of debates* in the process/project?

Operative planning and negotiating conflicts

We regard the operative planning as the process of doing and as a pragmatic discourse about social actions related to cognitive and pragmatic legitimacy. Social actions are created in an intersection between instrumental cost-benefit calculations and cultures characterized by cognitive models. Operative planning has the main purpose to advance pragmatic legitimacy and the power to implement what is democratic decided. Pragmatic legitimacy rests on self-interested actors who seek to maximize their utility. Achieving and maintaining this legitimacy requires actions that demonstrate both individual and collective benefits, is cognitive acceptable and fulfils the regulative purposes about the process being democratic, participative, fair, etc. When implementing actions, actors often use the standard solutions to the problems that have been successful before, and no other alternative is regarded as possible solution. The actors do not know any other way to act. This can be an appropriate action, but it is more likely that action is dominated of routines and the action can be a pervert respond to the problem. There is no learning at this level because the use of other standard operative procedures is instructed, and instructing is not defined as learning.

Operative planning includes the implementation of the production orders from the tactical planning, the planning of concrete measures and the daily implementation work. In local and regional planning, documents such as annual budgets, development plans, development contracts, etc. considered for operative planning.

Compared the term operative planning with Laverack and Labonte (2000) model of community capacity building, the term includes what they call strategy implementation and management. In Selznick (1957: 55–56) model of institutional leadership operative planning is to master internal conflicts that need to be sorted before the implementation of decided actions.

Based on our experiences operative planning is facing several challenges (Amdam, 2011):

- Lack of support from the institutional, strategic and tactical planning.
- Conflicting interest and uneven distributions of cost end benefits.
- Lack of commitment to the operative planning and the binding operative partnerships contracts.

The operative planning concerns discussion of the facts and data, and is a discourse linked to instrumental rationality and the pragmatic legitimacy. In a power perspective this involves having the knowledge and other resources to implement what has been politically decided, but it also involves preventing the implementation of such decisions. Operative planning refers to the local and regional capacity or power to implement planned action. A complete political will formation process with institutional, strategic, tactical and operative planning linked together can establish the necessary political legitimacy and power to implement actions at the operative level. Operative planning, which is separated from the other forms of planning, can easily meet strong resistance because it lacks regulative, normative and cognitive legitimate, even if the pragmatic legitimacy is high.

Operative planning is about putting plans into action and takes place in the space of action between the cognitively acceptable and the pragmatically useful. When plans are to be implemented in practice, cost-benefit assessments will always be an important assessment basis for both those who are in favour and those who are against the plan. The opposition can argue that the affected actors must deliver resources and cover costs without sufficient compensation, or they can argue against the plan because it simply involves changes in incorporated patterns of action. Therefore, the implementation of actions often requires an extensive coordination between the actors. We use *operative action plans* or *operative partnership contracts* as terms for these structures, and by this we understand agreements that legally regulate the actors' responsibilities for implementing the actions and changes. Instrumental rationality or synoptic planning can be a tool to accomplish these contracts of action, but normally synoptic planning requires an actor who has command power and full control over the implementation which is not the situation in collaborative planning.

When conflicts arise at operative level, the role of the process manager is to mediate the conflicts between the parties involved. Consequently, negotiation planning between equal actors will normally be the practical way of working to set up operative partnership contracts. According to Forester (2012) planners must therefore have skills that enable them to handle conflicts and establish action plans that determine who is to do what, why and when, thereby increasing the pragmatic legitimacy and the power to act. Consensus does not need to be the goal, but rather a situation in which one agrees to disagree, while yet being able to cooperate (agonism). If one regards HiAP as an implementation chain, negotiating these actions plans becomes institutional planning and the frame for the planning process at a lower governing level. Here the question of knowing why, what and how comes up again, but then in more limited processes that are anchored in the larger process that has clarified the questions on a more general level.

Operative public health planning must strengthen the pragmatic legitimacy and capacity for action to implement decisions. The idea here is that the institutional, strategic, tactical planning should contribute legitimacy to the operative planning so that democratic decisions can be carried out even if they meet some resistance. The people involved in HiAP will always assess their costs against the benefits they obtain from the processes and the plans. Thus, pragmatic legitimacy expresses the extent to which HiAP is regarded as useful and has the capacity to implement action.

These are self-evaluation questions that partners and manager of HiAP process/projects must ask themselves continuously about operative planning:

- How well is the question about implementation of HiAP activities addressed in the local/regional community?
- What actions have you as a partner or manager of HiAP process/project done to implemented actions in your organization and your community/district/county to promote better public health?
- How strong is the capacity of the process/project and the community/district/county to implement public health actions now?
- What new public health actions/projects are your process/project ready to implement?
- How do the planner/process manager execute the role as *mediator of conflicts* in the process/project?

Conclusion

HiAP approach is regarded as a multi-actor collaboration based on planning and partnership for the purpose of enabling people to increase their control over their health and its determinants. HiAP builds largely on the governance and communicative turn in the public sector and thus exists in the shadow of a vertical government structure with sectors, silos and a chain of command. In practice, HiAP challenges the established way of thinking and acting in the silos and tries to create a more holistic understanding and handling of problems and needs. To successfully involve different sectors and government levels in this work, HiAP requires strong democratic legitimacy and institutional capacity.

We have argued that a political will formation process with institutional, strategic, tactical and operative planning can maintain and increase HiAP's institutional capacity and democratic legitimacy. In this process, planning and evaluation is integrated in the process of knowing why, what, how and doing. However, since HiAP and other regional and local planning and development work is a continual process in which it is important to contribute to the various forms of legitimacy and capacity, we consider managing and monitoring as very important opportunities to promote a learning process at the different levels of planning and learning. Nevertheless, it is essential that the monitoring process, in addition to measuring measurable results instrumentally, also set the stage for broad participation and partnership building at the different levels in the planning and development work, that is institutional, strategic, tactic and operative level.

References

Agger, A. & Sørensen, E. 2018. Managing collaborative innovation in public bureaucracies. *Planning Theory*, 17 (1): 53–73. https://doi.org/10.1177/1473095216672500

Amdam, R. 2010. *Planning in Health Promotion Work: an Empowerment Model.* Abingdon, Oxon and New York: Routledge.

Amdam, R. 2011. *Planlegging og prosessleiing. Korleis lykkast i utviklingsarbeid.* Oslo: Samlaget.

Amdam, R. 2022: *Samskapt berekraft. Ei modell for samarbeidsdriven planlegging og innovasjon.* Rapport - nr. 115/2022. Volda: Høgskulen i Volda. https://bravo.hivolda.no/hivolda-xmlui/handle/11250/2991502

Amdam, R. 2023. "Health in all policies" in Norwegian municipalities—Dilemmas and lack of legitimacy and capacity. *International Journal of Health Planning and Management*, 38: 1345–1359. http://dx.doi.org/10.1002/hpm.3664

Amin, A. & Thrift, N. 1994. Living in the global. In: Amin, A. & Thrift, N. (eds.) *Globalization, Institutions, and Regional Development in Europe.* Oxford: Oxford University Press.

Ansell, C. & Gash, A. 2007. Collaborative governance in theory and practice. *Journal of Public Administration Research and Theory*, 18 (4): 543–571. https://doi:10.1093/jopart/mum032

Ansell, C. & Gash, A. 2012. Stewards, mediators, and catalysts: Toward a model of collaborative leadership. *The Innovation Journal: The Public Sector Innovation Journal*, 17(1): article 7. https://innovation.cc/wp-content/uploads/2012_17_1_7_ansell_gash_innovate-leadrship.pdf

Bache, I. & Olsson, J. 2001. Legitimacy through partnership? EU policy diffusion in Britain and Sweden. *Scandinavian Political Studies*, 24 (3): 215–237. https://doi.org/10.1111/1467-9477.00054

Bryson, J. M., Crosby, B. C. & Bloomberg, L. 2014. Public value governance: Moving beyond traditional public administration and new public management. *Public Administration Review*, 74 (4): 445–456. https://doi.org/10.1111/puar.12238

Etzioni, A. 1993. *The Spirit of Community: The Reinvention of American Society*. New York: Touchstone.

Etzioni 1988. *The Moral Dimension. Toward a New Economics*. London and New York: The Free Press.

Fetterman 2005. Empowerment evaluation principles in practice. In: Fetterman & Wandersman, D. M. (eds.) *Empowerment Evaluation Principles in Practice*. New York: Guilford Press.

Forester, J. 1993. *Critical Theory, Public Policy and Planning Practice: Toward a Critical Pragmatism*. Albany NY: University of New York Press.

Forester, J. 2012. On the theory and practice of critical pragmatism: Deliberative practice and creative negotiations. *Planning Theory*, 12(1): 5–22. https://doi.org/10.1177/1473095212448750

Gjertsen, A. & Halkier, H. 2004. Regional utvikling og partnerskap – et komparativt blikk på norske og danske erfaringer. In: Amdam, R. & Bukve, O. (eds.) *Det regionalpolitiske regimeskiftet – tilfellet Noreg*. Trondheim: Tapir Akademisk Forlag.

Healey, P. 1997. *Collaborative Planning. Shaping Places in Fragmented Societies*. London: Macmillan Press.

Healey, P. 1999. *Institutional Capacity-Building, Urban Planning and Urban Regenerating Projects*. Paper presented at the XII AESOP Congress. Aveiro: University of Aveiro. https://api.semanticscholar.org/CorpusID:112534533

Healey, P. 2005. Governance capacity, policy network, and territorial specificities. In: Albrechts, L. & Mandelbaum, S. J. (eds.) *The Network Society*. London: Routledge.

Langfield-Smith, K. & Smith, D. 2003. Management control systems and trust in outsourcing relationships. *Management Accounting Research*, 14: 281–307. https://doi.org/10.1016/S1044-5005(03)00046-5

Laverack, G. & Labonte, R. 2000. A planning framework for community empowerment goals within health promotion. *Health Policy and Planning*, 15, 3: 255–262. https://doi.org/10.1093/heapol/15.3.255

Lukes, S. 1974. *Power: A Radical View*. London: Macmillan.

Nicola, R. M. & Hatcher, M. T. 2000. A framework for building effective public health constituencies. *Public Health Management Practice*, 6 (2): 1–10. https://doi.org/10.1097/00124784-200006020-00003

Scott, W. R. 2002. *Organizations. Rational, Natural, and Open Systems*. 5th edition. London: Taylor and Francis.

Scott, W. R. 2014. *Institutions and Organizations: Ideas, Interests, and Identities*. *4th* edition. London: Sage Publications.

Selznick, P. 1957. *Leadership in Administration: A Sociological Interpretation*. New York: Harper and Row.

Sørensen, E. & Torfing, J. 2009. Making governance networks effective and democratic through metagovernance. *Public Administration*, 87 (2): 234–258. https://doi.org/10.1111/j.1467-9299.2009.01753.x

Sørensen, E. & Torfing, J. 2017. Metagoverning collaborative innovation in governance networks. *American Review of Public Administration*, 47 (7): 826–839. https://doi.org/10.1177/0275074016643181

Stoker, G. 1998. Governance as theory, five propositions. *Social Science Journal*, 50: 17–28. https://doi.org/10.1111/1468-2451.00106

Stoker, G. 2004. *Transforming Local Governance. From Thatcherism to New Labour*. London: Palgrave Macmillan.

Strand, T. 2001. *Ledelse, organisasjon og kultur*. Bergen: Fagbokforlaget.
Synnevåg, E. S., Amdam, R. & Fosse, E. M. 2018. Intersectoral planning for public health: Dilemmas and challenges. *International Journal of Health Policy and Management*, 7 (11): 982–992. https://doi.org/10.15171/ijhpm.2018.59
Tones, B. K. 1974. A systems approach to health education. *Community Health*, 6 (1): 34–40.
Tones, K. & Green, J. 2004. *Health Promotion*. London: Sage Publications.
Torfing, J. 2016. *Collaborative Innovation in Public Sector*. Washington DC: Georgetown University Press.
Torfing, J., Sørensen, E. & Røiseland, A. 2016. Transforming the public sector into arena for co-creation: Barriers, drivers, benefits, and the way forward. *Administration and Society*, 51 (5): 795–825. https://doi.org/10.1177/0095399716680057
Wilson, K. 2004. The complexities of multi-level governance in public health. *Canadian Journal of Public Health*, 95 (6): 409–412. https://doi.org/10.1007/bf03403981
World Health Organization. 2001. *Evaluation in Health Promotion. Principles and Perspectives*. WHO regional publications European series, No. 92. Geneva: World Health Organization. https://www.who.int/publications/i/item/9789289013598

6

REFLECTIONS

HiAP as a collaborative planning process

Achieving a high degree of democratic legitimacy for change is an important driving force in the public sector, but the question is whether HiAP in the form of public health planning and partnerships has sufficient political legitimacy and capacity to implement the wishes of the people and fulfil the purpose of public health policies. To discuss and answer this question this chapter uses the planning staircase in Chapter 5 to analyse data from one HiAP action research project (HEPRO), and research projects on HiAP in Norway before and during COVID-19.

Introduction

According to Nicola and Hatcher (2000) it is commonly recognized that public health work is about multi-actor and multilevel empowerment approaches including governmental policies and actions in the legal, economic and political arenas. It is about coalitions and inter-sectoral partnership between academic institutions, government agencies, NGOs and communities. Thus, building and sustaining formal and informal network organizations become necessary for maintaining relationship and communication channels. If public health leaders do not view networking as an ongoing and essential activity in the agency's operation, they may find that once useful communication channels no longer exist when they are needed. The key to successful network is identifying and assessing the network structure that is in place and understanding the effects of the structure on available resources in public health.

However, in the debate of methodology and methods there is still two paradigmatical positions. One is the traditional positivistic and instrumental approach that seeks causality between interventions and effects, and which inspire people to seek objective knowledge and quantitative evidence of effectiveness. The other

DOI: 10.4324/9781003451273-6

is the phenomenological and communicative approach which sees intervention as capacity-building process and regards subjective and qualitative information from the participants about their interpretation of the situation as valid data. In practice, the main question is how to combine the quantitative and qualitative methods, and therefore public health has a mix of methods as a typical character. In addition, public health work is ideologically committed to stimulate empowerment, which in its nature must be a balanced blend of instrumental and communicative rationalities. Hence, collaborative planning becomes relevant because evidence-based expert knowledge is combined with experience-based lay person knowledge in opinion and will making processes. This process can contribute to the capacity for action that can fight against, and potentially change the power of the hampering structuring forces. Somewhat simplistically, one can say that planning is understood both as an instrumental management process that emphasizes the design of the process and formal decision-making and control processes, and a communicative leadership process that emphasizes the relationships between people and how the actors learn from each other through communication, decisions and action.

One characteristic of empowered local and regional and communities is that extensive collaborative partnerships between the public, private and voluntary sectors exist both inside and outside the geographical territory. This does not mean that empowered local and regional communities are independent of instrumental power from the superior government and external enterprises, and that lagging local and regional communities are strongly dependent on support from the national government and external enterprises. In practice, all communities are dependent on a widespread interaction with their surroundings, but the balance of power can easily become asymmetric. The achievement of an appropriate balance of power between the communities and their surroundings is probably one of the most difficult tasks in local and regional development work. Both private enterprises and public governments can easily become too instrumental and top-down oriented, and thus send the communities into a *dependency relationship* (Friedmann, 1992; Friedmann & Weaver, 1979). This kind of dependency relationship can imply that actors outside the local and regional communities take important decisions and actions regarding the local and regional communities, and that people in the communities are not actively involved in the social learning and mobilizing process. In this way, the local and regional communities can enter a vicious circle that over time can weaken their own capability for facing new challenges, and get what can be called *local community AIDS* (Stöhr, 1990: 2).

Empowered local and regional communities have seemingly an administrative or a geographical limitation. But such a view misses out that these local and regional communities often are empowered and dynamic because they have both a territorial and a functional extent combined with a strong identity. This implies that one needs to consider the character of communities, such as history and context, when one designs local and regional planning and development interventions. Regional and local development is a slow, organic process. It takes root slowly and must be carefully nurtured before it begins to yield results. It must grow from within the local communities. However, planners who come from the outside can, among other things, help to develop a new self-understanding and improve their skills in self-help, direct action, negotiating and drawing up effective plans of action to achieve changes in policy processes and structures.

We argue that empowerment must be what Habermas (1996) calls a political will formation process substantiated in the form of collaborative planning that combines instrumental and communicative planning in local and regional communities and that mobilizes local and regional communities and enables the people to increase control over their health and its determinants. Habermas' (1996) will formation process has different discourses with their respective rationalities, and together, these form a political legitimizing and capacity-building process. The discursive processes are conducted by means of public argumentation. It is through the communicative process that actors become heard, influence each other and learn from each other. The actors develop relationships and both individual and collective capacity to act as actors with the power to influence current institutions and other structural forces. According to Giddens (1984), structure constrains agency, and agency alters structure over time. Hence, collaborative planning is a process in which the actors are influenced by structures like health determinants, but also a process in which the actors' actions are added together and become institutional structural forces. In this way, the collaborative process can change the determinants, rules, norms and beliefs embedded in institutions and thus pave the way for new actions and innovations.

However, the regional territorial and horizontal power is weak compared to the sectoral and vertical power in most of the western country's political power structure. The first is mainly a part of a territorial bottom-up governing system of governance partnerships, mobilization and competition between regions. The second is mainly a part of a top-down governing system dominated by government structure, sector-thinking, central planning and control of the welfare state production. It can be argued that the situation in general is a consequence of the modernization process in our societies (cf. Giddens, 1990). In this process instrumental rationality and top-down policy seem to dominate over the communicative rationality and bottom-up policy. Modern societies suffer under the instrumental rationalities and the neglect of communicative rationalities and collective processes. Habermas (1996) and Friedmann (1992) among others argue that the solution to the problem is to mobilize the territorial power to meet the sectoral power in a political process. In a regional and local policy context this means that the bottom-up and mainly communicative power can be used to equalize the top-down and mainly instrumental power and to build adequate local and regional development institutions.

In fact local and regional planning and development work more and more seem to take the form of a two-parallel system; (1) a government dominated, highly sectorized and single organization formal planning and (2) a governance-based spatial planning that tries to foster collaboration and partnership. Local and regional governance institutions are the key actors in the spatial planning, but they are often rather weak constructions that depend highly on the trust between the participants' willingness to collaborate, and their commitment to local and regional development. In practice, the bottom-up governance politics seems to depend on the top-down government politics.

Enhancing the local and regional capacity to take actions requires attention to decentralization, delegation and devolution, which, obviously must come in conflict with the political control and centralization prescribed by the economic organization theory (Christensen & Lægreid, 2004: 13; Lægreid & Rykkja, 2022). The growth of New Public Governance can therefore be regarded as a reaction to the structural forces of Traditional Public Administration and New Public Management, and the lack of accountability and increased fragmentation, silo-thinking and unit-selfishness that have been consequences of these governing systems. A major result of this politically intended development is that the state has ended up with less political power, and market forces and networks have gained more political power.

New Public Management reform is a worldwide process that makes public and voluntary organizations become more like private sector organizations with a dominance of instrumental rationality and internal focus. The New Public Management reforms seem to have freed managers from detailed political instructions but have not strengthened the political steering because of the lack of causality in the production of public sector services. In public sector production defining long-term and broadly accepted goals is difficult, and to establish obvious logical relations between input and outcome are challenging. In addition, the monitoring and management systems are so far more developed to handle *output* than *outcome* because the lack of knowledge about the causalities between the public sector activities and the results on the society. In addition, every activity and every effect that can be measured, tend to get most focus than other effects. Then the nearest solution could be more monitoring, more management and more accountability, but these activities do not solve the fundamental problem with the lack of causality in production of public sector services. When there is no obvious logical relation between a public sector organization activity or lack of activity, and the effects to the society, one cannot hold the organizations and their leaders responsible for the outcome and lack of outcome.

The New Public Management reforms have delegated power from the elected politicians to administrative leaders with the consequence that the politicians are not able to hold the public sector managers responsible for the outcome of the policy implementation, only the output. Now public and private sector leaders tend to be evaluated much the same way, that is by their ability to lead their organizations to perform measured by output indicators. This lack of *outcome accountability* gives the public sector managers the possibility to act in an egoistic way and makes it extremely difficult to obtain needed outcomes through the existing political and administrative sector structure, such outcomes as sustainable public health. When the silo-thinking is dominating, the potential outcomes from multi-actor collaboration always will be compared with the transaction coast of staying in contact with the partners. The basic question for the participants seems to be *what is in it for me* as a partner. Therefore, the reforms and the fragmentation of the political power structure have reduced the public sector's ability and willingness to participate in network organizations because the leaders have become more focused on internal issues and their production of outputs than the external effects. Today the politicians get blamed when people do not like the outcome of public sector production, but the politicians are not able to hold the public sector managers responsible for the outcome of the policy implementation, only the output.

In addition, when the lack of outcome accountability gives the public sector organizations the possibility to act in an egoistic way, it becomes extremely difficult to realize local and regional territorial planning and development through governance and network organizations that require altruistic actions. This situation can reduce the existing and potential power of local and regional governance and partnership activity because the creations of these are very dependent on trust between the participants and willingness to support the production of common good. If one regards governance as a response to the fragmentation of the state, and if the government institutions have become more egoistic, Jessop (1997) may be correct when he writes that governance still seems to exist in the shadow of government.

As far as we can draw conclusions from our discussion, there seems to be a similar governance turn in public health work and the experiences from this turn seem to be similar to the experiences from regional politics. A common and overall experience is that governance is a complicated process. To make a territorial counterforce to the sectorized power that dominates modern societies, partnerships in public health as well as other local and regional development, need to create legitimacy from inside the community and achieve acceptance and legitimacy from outside. But this conclusion implies that HiAP is facing a dilemma. Partnerships within the governance structure need to be strong enough to influence their partners from the government structure but is that possible in governance-based partnerships where the participants from the government structure are free to leave. Handling this dilemma is at the core of what HiAP as policymaking is about.

HiAP represents a collaborative approach that articulates health considerations and integrates them into policymaking, both vertically within different government authorities and horizontally between the public, private and voluntary sectors, with the mission to improve the health of all communities and all people (Ståhl et al., 2006). Hence, HiAP, planning and politics are about power, and in democracy the use of power must be legitimate. Public health planning and partnerships need democratic legitimacy and institutional capacity, which refers to the legitimacy created by decisions that reflect the will of the people.

For HiAP the great challenge is how to combine the conventional and instrumental discourse with the communicative discourse in the practice of planning, participation, partnership, and policymaking. This challenge can be understood as a result of the modernization of the society and the need for a better balance between instrumental and communicative rationalities. In the modernization process instrumental rationality and top-down policy seem to dominate over the communicative rationality and bottom-up policy. When this modern logic becomes dominant, strong professions and their respective sector authorities, who base their existence on mainly instrumental rationality, can achieve a strong position in the society. Therefore, there is a strong need for cross-sector networking and public sector managers are expected to take part in partnerships and collaborative local and regional planning and development at the same time as public sector organizations have become more instrumental, out-put-oriented, silo-structured and unit-egoistic.

In Chapter 1 we ended the introduction with stating demands about what HiAP must contribute to. In the following chapters these demands have been nuanced, and we have argued that HiAP must become radical New Public Governance, a political will formation process which can be designed as collaborative planning and as a process of knowing why, what, how and doing. Thus, the demands in Chapter 1 must be reformulated to *questions*:

- About knowing why: The demand that HiAP must contribute to increased legitimacy (outcomes/impacts), must be supplemented with the question does institutional planning increase HiAP's regulative legitimacy and the power to design and setting frames for the process?
- About knowing what: The demand that HiAP must contribute to increased quality (outcomes/impacts), must be supplemented with the question does strategic planning increase HiAP's normative and regulative legitimacy and the power to set the agenda?
- About knowing how: The demand that HiAP must contribute to increased effectiveness (outcomes/results), must be supplemented with the question does tactical planning increase HiAP's regulative and cognitive legitimacy and the capacity to make decisions?
- About doing: The demand that HiAP must contribute to increased production and efficiency (outputs), must be supplemented with the question does operative planning increase HiAP's cognitive and pragmatic legitimacy and the capacity of doing?

Managing and monitoring the HEPRO project

The main goal of the HEPRO project was to integrate health considerations into spatial planning and development and to make an important contribution to a sustainable public health policy in Europe (see Textbox 6.1). HEPRO consisted of 32 partners and brought together people with expert and specialist knowledge and experience

TEXTBOX 6.1 ABOUT HEPRO

Along with the rest of Europe, the BSR is facing enormous health challenges. An ageing population, migration of young people from rural areas to the cities, unemployment, increase in alcohol and drug abuse, mental illness and lifestyle diseases especially contribute to these challenges.

They require imaginative, complex and diverse solutions. A solution must have its focus not only at risk factors, but also on factors that are positive and promote health conditions for the individuals. We call a broad inter-sectoral effort like this "The New Public Health effort".

The HEPRO project was running as a public health project in 2005–2008 and was part financed by EU in the BSR INTERREG IIIB programme. The national Healthy Cities networks in the BSR were initiative-takers and HEPRO was professionally supported by the World Health Organization (WHO). The WHO Healthy Cities approach seeks to put health high on the political and social agenda of cities, and to build a strong movement for public health at the local level. The HEPRO concept is underpinned by the principles of the WHO Health for All strategy and Local Agenda 21.

HEPRO is characterized by:

- A system theoretical approach to policy production
- A circular and communicative understanding of planning
- A spatial and cross-sectoral focus on public health

HEPRO aimed to integrate health consideration into spatial planning and development.

Strong emphasis was given to empowerment; including equity, participatory governance and solidarity, inter-sectoral collaboration and action to address the determinants of health.

Furthermore, the project aimed at making an important contribution to a sustainable public health policy in Europe. The HEPRO planning model is also a part of the work with quality development within the public health field.

Among the results from the project are the HEPRO planning model, the HEPRO survey model, a questionnaire which was answered by 33,000 respondents in the BSR, an interactive webpage and a database of results for future research purposes. In line with the vision of HEPRO the project will be followed up by a new project which builds, among others, upon the results and experiences obtained in HEPRO.

We hope that this publication will both inform and inspire towards further work within the HEPRO goal: increased focus on health and well-being in the Baltic Sea Region.

Source: Wangberg and Dyrseth (2008:5), printed in Amdam (2010: 86).

from all relevant sectors across 8 countries around the Baltic Sea Region (BSR). The project should help sharing effective ways to promote health and bring the results to attention to those who need to act. The project should carry out a transnational population survey and training programmes and implement concrete findings from the survey into the spatial planning processes (Østfold County Council, 2005: 4).

The HEPRO planning model represented a systematic and comprehensive long-term approach to public health planning in the communities. The aim was to show step by step how a plan where health and well-being aspect is highlighted can be carried out and embedded in the ordinary planning in the municipality/county/district. The model was a systematic approach in six steps linked together in a circle with a dynamic character. The circle followed a planning period of four years. The six steps were (Østfold County Council, 2005: 5): attention, insight and new knowledge, building a platform for joint action, implementation, documentation and evaluation. This last step in the planning circle was an evaluation of structure, process and results and the evaluation should give input to the starting point for a new planning circle. HEPRO's planning model was shown in the project overview as a circular model where each step follows the other (Østfold County Council, 2005). The planning approach should be based on empowerment and should contribute to self-development, participatory governance, solidarity, cross-sectoral cooperation and action and consider important factors that affect health (Østfold County Council, 2005: 4; Amdam, 2010).

The project was audited by EU, and in the New Public Management tradition the project was kept accountable mostly for implementing the planned activities and keeping the project within the budget. There was no formal evaluation at the end of the project that could clarify to what extent the project had reached its goals. What we can say about the goals on *output* is that the survey of the population's state of health was successfully completed and the data were used across the national boundaries, and a training programme in public health work and local health profiles became integrated parts of the project. In addition, health profiles and environmental factors related to health have been used as a basis for a public health policy at local and regional level. When it comes to the goals on outcome and impacts, we only have the collected midways data about how the partners evaluated the situation at that time.

When we asked the partners what are the most important outputs and the most significant outcomes/impacts on the public health situation from the public health project so far, they answered:

- Difficult to say what the results of our activities are and what the results of other social, cultural and economic factors within the family, the neighbourhood, the workplace, etc. are.
- Expect the most significant outcomes to come from the results of the health survey.

To collect data about the process and the output is normally an easy part of the documentation, but to get data about the outcomes and impacts on the public health work is a far more demanding and complicated. Therefore, there seem in project like the HEPRO project, to be a bias towards reporting the easily collected data about the outputs and neglecting the more difficult data about the outcomes and impacts. This lack of data has consequences for the learning process because there is a need for data about the outcomes and impacts of the intervention to legitimate the public health work, keep it on the political agenda, involve more people and enforce the capacity to handle public health issues.

The doings. Operative planning, pragmatic legitimacy and power to implement

Some self-reported activities and outputs from the HEPRO partners concerning operative planning are listed in Textbox 6.2.

TEXTBOX 6.2 SELF-REPORTED ACTIVITIES AND OUTPUTS FROM THE HEPRO

- Educating the employees of the municipality in collaboration with local educational institutes.
- Activities for employees: "Training creates well-being" and a "training group to prevent sickness".
- In collaboration with a college, the public health servants have been offered courses in health promotion.
- Training programmes/education and seminars about public health for local municipality employees, employees of own organization, school nurses, family doctors and for public in general etc.
- Forums to citizens to participate and involve, stimulation to participation in community development (children and youths are especially prioritised).
- Health promoting school regional centre works with schools and youth.
- Health centre realized seminars for school nurses, family doctors.
- Actions aimed at vulnerable groups and individuals; youth health centres, guidance groups for parents and pregnant women, facilitated physical training for the elderly, integrating handicapped people, programme for alcoholism and drug abuse.
- Welfare department has cooperation with NGO "Youth federation", to provide social work on streets of the city.
- Daily centre for persons with mental disabilities.
- Developing sports, outdoor activity, walking and bicycling possibilities and activities.

- Social meeting places to prevent isolation and loneliness.
- Support of and collaboration with voluntary charity organizations.
- No smoking in all public workplaces from the first of January 2007.
- Education in the public schools.
- Results and experiences summarised through predetermined evaluation reports.
- Environmental certification stimulates to learning through regular evaluations.

Source: Amdam (2010: 97–99)

The implemented activities that are listed in Textbox 6.2 show that there are a lot of activities that can contribute to personal and local empowerment and capacity building, and these activities indicate that the overall goal of the project, empowerment and personal and collective capacity building, is accepted and implemented. Many of these activities have potential outputs and outcomes that can contribute to the learning at tactical and operative level, but the outputs and outcomes on strategic and institutional planning are more diffuse. One of the main questions that have to be raised in that respect, is to what extent the project has improved the HEPRO partners capacity to handle health promotion and prevention issues, and to what extent the process has contributed to empowerment of individuals and communities.

Knowing how. Tactical planning, cognitive legitimacy and power to decide

Some self-reported activities from the HEPRO partners concerning tactical planning are listed in Textbox 6.3. According to these activities the HEPRO partners have been mobilizing resources, networking, organizing, planning and integrating public health perspective in the daily work. When we asked our HEPRO partners about the challenges they are facing, they answered that project represents a new organization at that there is a lack of human resources. The common answer was that the direct responsibility for the public health often went to only one person, the project leader and often he/she was a coordinator of many public health projects. The project leaders reported that they had problems with finding time to prioritize the work and to find proper areas for collaboration. The HEPRO partners reported that the main challenge was to work out health policies with strong involvement of professionals and citizens. They reported a need for increased competence among the different professions but could already in the middle of the project see some increased political and administrative capacity to handle the health promotion work.

We interpret the reported activities so that, in sum, they are more likely to be considered conservative co-productions than radical co-creations. This means that

TEXTBOX 6.3 SELF-REPORTED ACTIVITIES FROM THE HEPRO PARTNERS CONCERNING TACTICAL PLANNING

- Developed a political and administrative structure concerning promotion of health issues and preventive issues, which will be the carrying capacity in regards of solving the present and future assignments.
- Close cooperation to the public health service suppliers.
- Deeper and more active cooperation of public health sector and municipality administration and council.
- Involvement of politicians and representatives of municipality administration to public health discussions.
- Health Impact Assessment using as a tool when making political decisions.
- Health and environmental consequences assessment of all proposals, in the physical planning, in political decisions.
- A cheque list to ensure that public health has focus in all planning.
- Environmental management system (ISO 14001) – community works for certification in 2007.
- Working on a plan for our environment that also includes a health focus.
- Concept clarification of the broad health and environment concept in the physical planning.
- Networking: cross-sectoral and multidisciplinary co-operation – such as healthcare professionals, planners, social advisers, economists.
- Cooperation with State Agency Health promoting centre taking a part in their public activities, giving customs free places for activities realising and in every day work by using materials from Centre – booklets, posters.
- Carrying out different training programmes, site visits among partners, also exchanging experts in public health and other health related matters.
- Encouraging organizations to create public health projects.
- New public health measures are adopted as part of the activity and economy plans for the coming year and budgets.
- Public health initiatives are given priority and are funded as part of the annual plans.
- Creation of organizations and centres of preventive activities.
- Established a Health Centre that should ensure a direct contact between the professional environment and the citizens with chronic diseases.
- Organized projects in collaboration with voluntary charity organizations and/or the county.
- Encouraged NGOs to do public health initiatives and organize activities.

Source: Amdam (2010: 96)

their purpose was to bring about cooperation between actors from different levels and sectors within the established government structure. There are few if any activities that clearly show that the purpose was to challenge the current power structure to work and organize in a completely new way so that the partnerships can be considered radical co-creation where the partners manage to define problems and solutions in completely new ways, and not just as a compromise between the partners' incorporated ways of working.

Knowing what. Strategic planning, normative legitimacy and power to set political agenda

Some self-reported activities from the HEPRO partners about what they have done concerning strategic planning are listed in Textbox 6.4.

TEXTBOX 6.4 SELF-REPORTED ACTIVITIES FROM THE HEPRO PARTNERS ABOUT WHAT THEY HAVE DONE CONCERNING STRATEGIC PLANNING

- Involving citizens in development and implementation of the policy on health.
- Managed to get health on the political agenda, including a political decision to form a health project committee.
- Use of information and data from HEPRO survey for the formation of public health strategy/health promotion and prevention plan and other activities.
- Informed politicians and decision-makers and general population information about health status of the municipality.
- Theme days regarding the result of the health profile, together with the local forum, the political dialog committee, the political subcommittees, project committees and the administrative organization, the voluntary societies and the collaboration partners on the health areas.
- Involving the politicians and placing the health projects on the political agenda, establishing a health prize, campaigns, for example press campaigns.
- Keep health issues on the politician's agenda, through initiation of a number of activities, most of them are and will be based upon citizen involvement strategies.
- Site visits, study trips and meetings regarding health promotion and prevention in HEPRO context, where politicians and the decision-makers participated.

- A campaign to promote citizen involvement in as well the making as the realization of a municipal health policy.
- Relate people to planning and plan documents via communications and dialogue, e.g. contacts via municipal services (the strategy has been educating the public servants and rewarding relevant efforts), contact with the voluntary charitable organizations (the strategy has been economic and practical support of activities), public participation in municipal planning.

Source: Amdam (2010: 94–95)

In the HEPRO project, a survey of public health in the various partner countries was a large and important part of the project, and it appears from the self-reporting that these surveys are used actively by the partners. The lesson we draw from this is that register data and questionnaire surveys can be an important tool for gaining insight into the public health situation in various local communities and regions. A survey gives a lot of different data about how people regard their situation and what impact the public health work and other factors have on their situation. However, the data needs to be analysed and interpreted if they shall be used in the planning and policymaking process. In addition, there is a need for involving people in the dialogs between the experts and politicians to make a common understanding of what problems that need to be solved first and how people can contribute to solving the problems. The creation of this common understanding and the mobilization of people and their resources can increase the local and regional capacity to handle the public health problems that are mapped in the survey.

From the answers we can read that the empowerment planning approach is understood and used. Broad participation is reported as important tools in the problem assessment and interpretation, and a main goal for the strategic planning is to put health promotion on the political agenda and to include health promotion activities in the planning documents. These answers seem to confirm the experience from other action research on the local and regional planning, that people easily get mobilized in the discussion of strategic issues that concern them, but in the policymaking process there is a critical stage between the discussion and the actual involvement in organizations that can implement actions (Amdam, 2011).

Knowing why. Institutional planning, regulative legitimacy and power to setting frames

Some self-reported activities from the HEPRO partners concerning institutional planning and increased regulative legitimacy and capacity to design processes are listed in Textbox 6.5.

TEXTBOX 6.5 SELF-REPORTED ACTIVITIES FROM THE HEPRO PARTNERS CONCERNING INSTITUTIONAL PLANNING

- Meetings, talks, discussions, reflections about health, personal and professional values.
- Dissemination of public health information though newspapers and internet.
- Collaboration with HEPRO project, Healthy Cities Network, etc.
- HEPRO project has created a background for the development of public health activities through EU support and local projects.
- Being at the starting point, and the most significant impacts of the health project so far have been the high level of attention.
- National Institute for Health Development finances local activities.
- Structural reform in Denmark that gives an opportunity to build up the health area from ground.
- Established a steering group, forum for Public Health, etc. including politicians, health planers, health promoters and health chief represented to follow the process. Established different political subcommittees, to reassure the spatial healthy planning.
- A working group on public health and sustainable development work, e.g. including the local districts leading medical doctor, the leader of the child and school health clinic, coordinator for crime prevention, the environmental health expert, the local urban planner and the Local Agenda 21-coordinator.
- Especially efforts to involve the politicians in order they would have more interest in public health problems.
- Politicians in our municipality have passed the budget for 2007 with 1.1 million Euros for activities.
- Collaboration with other organizations and institutions, etc. organized through participation in different networks.
- The composition of health plans which covers all areas of politics in community, e.g. utilising the results from the health survey. Close involvement of decision-makers, politicians, citizens and different organizations (NGOs etc.).
- Spread of information on HEPRO-project activity and future possibilities. Spreading the information through different channels.
- Networking is a tool to create involvement among citizens.

Source: Amdam (2010: 100–101)

As planning expert and advisor in the process, we clarified that the various phases in the planning circle must not come in a fixed order. This is because we believe that planning, policymaking, and institution building is a continuous but not linear process. Concretely, this means that in a project such as HEPRO, the implementation of a health activity can take place at the same time as the work to create awareness and to put another health activity on the political agenda. We further said that when the circle is used as a metaphor, it is important to understand that after one round in the circle the participants are not back in the situation where they started. The situation will have changed, and those involved have, among other things, learned what works and what doesn't, what is easy to implement and what meets resistance. The answers indicate that this circular planning process is understood and adapted, at least by some of the partners. However, we must have in mind that the partners gave these answers in the middle of the project.

We have learned that it is important to emphasize that development can be intensified by way of a project, but that regional and local community development is nonetheless a continuous process. In our advices to the HEPRO project we therefore said that the project must be understood as an intervention in a continuous public health work process, and therefore the project must carry out activities in cooperation with regional and local partners when they are ready to participate, and not wait with all the activities until action programmes are decided. Normally these action programmes require institutional partnerships between actors which can commit themselves to governance networks. The HEPRO partners solved this issue differently, some partners worked more communicatively than others.

We based our advises on the ISTOL-model and maintained that the purpose was to increase the local and regional capacity to manage public health in an appropriate balance between top-down and bottom-up policies. It was further assumed that there were no simple answers to how to balance top-down and bottom-up policy, and that the combination had to be designed in the actual situation and context. The implication of this understanding was that the project should contribute to the partners gaining a better ability to manage themselves, focus on their challenges, implement actions and learn from their experiences. In order to get an indication of the HEPRO project as a continuous process, we can look at what the partners answered when we asked them about whom in the organization and the community/district/county have learned about public health so far, what have they learned and how is this learning expressed in the public health work?

- The politicians in the health committee and the chief of the health department have learned that prevention and health promotion is a very important overriding value and that a comprehensive effort is necessary.
- Municipal organization public servants and professional groups have learned more about the relationship between physical and social environmental factors, health and well-being.

- In society, there is reason to suggest that knowledge about healthy habits and a health-promoting lifestyle have increased among the municipality's children and youths.

The activities at institutional level tell us that being a partner in the HEPRO project has given the local public health work regulative legitimacy, and that the partners used this legitimacy as a platform for cross-sector collaboration, networking, organizing, participation, etc. in order to get the health promotion and prevention more accepted and legitimized.

We concluded that project had moved the different partners in direction of fulfilling the goals of the project (Amdam, 2010). However, there were great differences between the partners on how they interpreted and implemented the project. There seemed to be a systematic difference between the western and eastern European partners. Communicative rationality, broad participation and bottom-up policymaking in the public health work, seemed to be far more accepted in the Nordic countries, compared to, for example, Poland. In the case from Denmark, the process was bottom-up oriented and very communicative. In the case from Poland, the planning is top-down and expert dominated, and very instrumental in the planning approach. In the Poland case, there seemed to be a lack of trust between the experts and the people. We can add that when the survey data was collected the survey was sent by mail to and from the respondents in the western European partners but had to be collected through personal interviews in the eastern European countries. Svendsen and Svendsen (2006) have compared the social capital in Denmark and Poland, and have found a much stronger trust among people and a stronger trust to the countries' political institutions in Denmark than in Poland. We find it plausible that the differences of social capital and trust in the two countries can explain the great differences between the two partners in how they interpreted and implemented the HEPRO project.

According to the ISTOL-model our main advice to the HEPRO project partners was that planning as an institutional, strategic, tactical and operative activity that should influence different capacity variables and contribute to various forms of legitimacy, and that stimulating the weak variables was the most important thing to succeed with the capacity-building process. As we interpret the reporting, the HEPRO project has contributed to increasing local and regional capacity to work with public health. But when we look at production and the results from the process, there are big differences between the partners. Some of the differences can be explained by how and under what conditions the process was implemented. In countries with highly centralized political power and strong respect for planners as experts, there seems to be little room for communicative forms of planning, broad participation and bottom-up politics. In these countries, the legitimacy of the local and regional public health work depends to a decisive extent on the legitimacy that the national authorities give to the work.

HiAP in the county of Møre and Romsdal before and during COVID-19

Introduction

Norway has around 5.5 million inhabitants and is a country with a challenging topography when it comes to providing the whole country with equal public services. The country has over 40 public hospitals with a local hospital function for the residents in their area, over 10 smaller public hospitals and around 10 private hospitals without a local hospital function. The public hospitals are organized into 20 health trust with their own boards. These trusts are subordinated to one of four regional health authorities, which also have their own boards. In Møre and Romsdal county, there are four hospitals organized in Møre and Romsdal Health Trust (MRHT) and subordinated to the Mid-Norway Regional Health Authority. The hospitals are responsible for the specialist health services. Furthermore, the country is divided into 15 county municipalities and 357 municipalities. The largest municipality has over 700,000 inhabitants and the smallest a few hundred inhabitants. Møre and Romsdal county has 27 municipalities. The municipalities are responsible for the primary health services and the public health. See Textbox 6.6.

TEXTBOX 6.6 A PRESENTATION OF MØRE AND ROMSDAL COUNTY

Møre and Romsdal county is located in North-West Norway between Vestland and Trøndelag and borders the Norwegian Sea in the north-west and Innlandet in the south-east. At the beginning of 2023, the population was 266,365, and the county has a land area of 13,840 km^2. In the last ten years, the population has increased by just over 4%, which is lower than the country. The population composition is changing. In 2022, for the first time, more people died than were born in Møre and Romsdal.

The county is divided into three regions, Sunnmøre, Romsdal and Nordmøre, and after changes in boundaries and municipal structure in 2019 and 2020, there was a decrease from 36 to 26 municipalities. Demographically, there are relatively large differences in population between the municipalities, and many of them are small. Topographically, the county is a typical West-Norway county, with fjords, mountains and islands, but where larger parts of the mountains have a more alpine feel than elsewhere in the country. The topography means that there are a number of natural hazards. Møre and Romsdal is the most landslide-prone county in the country, and one of the few counties that may be at risk of experiencing several major landslides. Throughout history, several large landslides have been highly destructive and led to tidal waves that have claimed many lives. There is a situation around Åkerneset in Storfjorden, a rock-dangerous mountain area that is classified as a high-risk site for large landslides which can cause a tidal wave that would have major consequences for the residential area along the fjord.

The county can otherwise experience a lot of weather, particularly affecting the sea in the north-west – and strong winds and rainfall are not unusual. Extreme weather in the form of storms and hurricanes is what leads to the most damages of natural phenomena in Norway, and Møre and Romsdal has had several incidents, such as the New Year's hurricane in 1992 and the extreme weather Dagmar in 2011. Another recent incident occurred on Hustadvika in 2019, when the cruise ship "Viking Sky" with more than 1,300 people on board had an engine failure and was close to running aground in bad weather conditions.

This backdrop has something to do with how preparedness is viewed in the county, and there has traditionally been a high focus on preparedness. In the knowledge base for the new planning strategy towards 2030 for Møre and Romsdal, it is stated that the county is a "laboratory for social security and preparedness". The actors from the emergency services (police, health, fire) and the administration have regular exercises, and a successful handling of the "Viking Sky" accident the year before the pandemic broke out in full, demonstrated that many years of joint training and interaction have worked. The interaction between different actors and levels of administration has also played an important and decisive role in the handling of the pandemic in Møre and Romsdal, and how to manage crisis cooperation in the county.

Source: Amdam et al. (2025 work in progress)
(Our translation from Norwegian to English)

The trusts and municipalities have a large degree of local autonomy, and the coordination of the health services is difficult because the health trusts and the municipalities have different management lines. The health trust and the specialist health services have a state management line with professional boards, and the primary health services have a municipal management line with elected local politicians. (Nylenna, 2014). A collaborative reform called the *Coordination Reform* was established in 2012 to connect the two management lines more closely both organizationally and financially. The purpose was to develop a greater degree of equality and partnership thinking and the ability to make binding consensus-based decisions (Ministry of Health and Care, 2019). In evaluations of the Coordination Reform, it is found that both the health trusts and the municipalities feel that the assignments of responsibility to the municipalities have become more complex and that it does not correspond to available resources (Rohde et al., 2020). One consequence of this is that providing health services becomes essential and prioritized, and that prevention and early intervention in public health have been de-prioritized, which can result in more hospital admissions (Rommetvedt & Nødland, 2020). The reform and the established collaboration agreements are nevertheless perceived as necessary tools, but they have not contributed to significantly more equality between the health company and the municipalities, which has been a central ambition in the Coordination Reform (Rommetvedt, 2021).

Regarding HiAP in municipalities and county municipalities, we have done a narrative review of HiAP in Norway (Amdam, 2023). Norwegian municipalities have for a long time carried out public health work, both as health promotion and health prevention. The municipalities have been partners in national public health programmes for a long time. Our conclusion is that HiAP so far has not generated enough political power to influence policy in the various sectors and at the various government levels, something on which public health work depends to succeed. The planning process does not function as a complete policy legitimizing and capacity-building process in which the various forms of planning, such as frame setting, communicative planning, coordinative planning and traditional rational planning, stimulate the various forms of legitimacy, especially normative and cognitive legitimacy. For HiAP, lack of legitimacy implies weak action capacity and problems in the accomplishment of its mission: empowering people to take more responsibility for their own health.

Our conclusion gets support from an investigation by the Office of the Auditor General (2015) which assessed the extent to which public health work in the municipalities and county municipalities is systematic and long term in scope, as well as how government instruments support public health work locally and regionally. Its main findings were:

- Most municipalities have not established systematic public health work.
- Work with public health and public health measures is not sufficiently knowledge based.
- Public health work is not sufficiently well anchored in sectors outside of health.
- There is a need to strengthen the follow-up on municipal public health work.

In addition, the investigation uncovered wide variation among municipalities and a need for more long-term and more systematic public health work and for more attention to general preventive measures.

In general, Norway was little prepared for the COVID-19 pandemic (Official Norwegian Report, 2021: 6, 2022: 5, 2023: 16). Lund-Tønnesen and Christensen (2023) have studied what national governing authorities in Norway have learned from pandemic management, and the investigation points to the fact that coordination is challenging, and that having the capacity to carry out analyses and to inform about strict restrictions is important. However, Christensen and Lægreid (2023a) found that the political leadership at national level succeeded rather well with connecting governance capacity and legitimacy in a co-production process with the public, and they write: "The government was able to make sense of the unfolding situation and to collaborate across administrative levels, policy areas, and sectors. Fundamental political decisions were not delegated to experts and professionals alone but were taken in collaboration, thus enhancing the ability to make sense of the situation as it unfolded" (Christensen & Lægreid, 2023a: 778).

There is a lot of research on the interaction at national level during the COVID-19 pandemic (for instance Capano et al., 2020; Christensen & Lægreid, 2022a) but very little at local and regional level. We have therefore participated in a research project whose purpose was to study pandemic management in Møre and Romsdal county, and was entitled "Before, during and after the pandemic: What lessons can specialist and municipal health services and users take away from the interaction about COVID-19?" Publishing the results from this project is in progress. In this chapter, we want to investigate whether the conclusions from research at national level in Norway about HiAP applies at regional and local level in Møre and Romsdal county regarding the interaction between health trusts and municipalities, and the handling of COVID-19 (Amdam et al. 2025).

The doings. Operative planning – pragmatic legitimacy and power to implement decisions

The narrative review showed that HiAP is confronted with strong political expectations to creating action because one expects benefit from the work, and because the benefit of prevention is always assessed against the benefit of meeting urgent needs. Thus, many municipalities have seen the advantages of participating in national programmes to carrying out activities. In this work, the municipalities cooperate more with the county and the ministries, than with the hospital trusts which in general have little connection to this work (Amdam, 2023). But for both the municipalities and the hospitals, health service is by far the most comprehensive activity, and the cooperation between the trusts and the municipalities is characterized by specific discussions about the municipal obligation to pay for patients ready for discharge from the hospitals, and the lack of resources for the assigned health service.

When the pandemic came, the MRHT and the municipalities quickly saw the need to put in place testing and diagnosis of employees and patients as well as the general population in the county. During the pandemic, the municipalities had a great responsibility to vaccinate, test, prevent infection, track infection, inform, etc., and the municipalities played a key role in handling the pandemic at local level and that the pandemic was handled effectively.

Both in MRHT and the municipalities, internal information flow and informing the population were prioritized in the day-to-day work with the pandemic. The employees could link up to various information channels and discussion forums so that they could always be well updated. Furthermore, the user committee at the MRHT took on an important role as a provider of information to its users during the pandemic.

In summary, we can say that at the operative level, the pragmatic discussions before the pandemic were characterized by conflicts about co-productions and the cost and benefits of hospitals' specialist services and the municipalities' primary services. During the pandemic, this changed radically. With few exceptions, everyone saw the benefit of a broad public health effort that could handle the pandemic, and the benefit of collaboration between municipalities, the MRHT and other governing bodies regarding health prevention, health promotion and health services. Here it must be added that the population's response to and cooperation on the crisis measures was great and decisive for the outcome. This gave the crisis management great pragmatic legitimacy and the capacity to carry out decisions. One can therefore say that HiAP had far more pragmatic legitimacy and capacity to implement activities during the pandemic than before the pandemic. The work was both task-focused and solution-oriented. The individual and collective benefits of the measures during the pandemic were assessed as great by both the municipalities, MRHT and not least the population.

Knowing how. Tactical planning, cognitive legitimacy and power to make decisions

The narrative review of HiAP in Norway showed a weak link between public health work's activities and the municipal's budgets and spatial plans, and the interests that promote growth and development seem to be stronger than those interests that promote public health. The review also showed that public health work is closely linked to the health sector and that the sector has difficulties in establishing cooperation with other sectors. In the municipalities, a cognitive understanding has taken hold that public health work belongs to the health sector's area of responsibility, this even though HiAP says the opposite (Amdam, 2023).

A major tactical debate in Norway has been about location, amalgamation and organization of health services in relation to equal access to services. This has also been discussed in the collaboration between MRHT and the municipalities, but the debate has especially been linked to assigned new tasks and insufficient funding, and the reallocation of some hospital health services. Our investigation in Møre and Romsdal showed that the cooperation between the municipalities and MRHT was characterized by formalized processes and the expert knowledge of the hospital doctors. The municipalities had to mobilize and cooperate if they were to establish countervailing power to this expertise, and MRHT regraded the municipalities as strong when they stood together on issues, and when it came to adopting the collaboration agreements politically. In general, the processes were formalized, and the autonomy of the actors challenged the decision-making power in the collaboration. The debate about getting to compromises about how to co-produce health services have been hampered because of the actors' formal legal and financial framework.

During the pandemic, the national and local cognitive legitimacy was challenged by the ethical dilemma of whether the governing authorities could order health workers to expose themselves to danger by working with corona patients, and whether the governing authorities could order health workers to vaccinate. For the employees, the question was how much the governing bodies through law and regulations could force them to act contrary to the norms and standards of the profession and their own values, needs and interests. These are examples of typical ethical dilemmas that do not only arise in crisis situations but are widely known and are discussed in the country and internationally. In crisis situations, it may be necessary to handle ethical dilemmas differently than in a normal situation, but none of our informants in Møre and Romsdal county highlight ethical conflicts that greatly hinder the handling of the pandemic in the county and the municipalities.

To handle the tasks that came with COVID-19, MRHT and the municipalities organized the collaboration through a new structure that was modelled after the agreed formal structure from 2015 as part of the Coordination Reform. The agreement and the formal structure became less important, and an informal structure was established with a Monday meeting for the county together, and with a Tuesday/Wednesday meeting for the four local hospital areas. These meeting were digital and could have over 100 participants, nevertheless the meeting seems to have functioned as face-to-face dialogues. The informal structure had a more limited participation than the formal structure demanded, but the collaboration activated many doctors, and the meetings contributed to effective decision-making processes. The professionals' assessments and actions became important in the decision-making processes.

The collaboration process during COVID-19 seems to have been characterized by common understanding and ability to make changes because the pandemic demanded action and quick results. Regular dialogue meetings were quickly established with key actors who ensured that there was a common understanding of the situation and that one was moving in the same direction. Our analysis indicated that the actors during COVID-19, experienced being more equal and mutually dependent, and with a strong motivation to fight the pandemic together.

MRHT and the municipalities showed an ability to take joint decisions, often on the advice of the professional representatives. They were quick to establish crisis management, and in the municipalities the municipal chief doctors were given a central role in decision-making. Cooperation which was met with resistance before the pandemic, was now adopted and carried out. The actors tried to stay within the legal frames, but to find good local solutions they stretched the boundaries of what was previously considered acceptable by the participating actors. In this way, crisis management in the county gained both high cognitive legitimacy and the capacity to make decisions.

Knowing what. Strategic planning, normative legitimacy and power to set the agenda

The narrative review of HiAP in Norway showed that HiAP is largely dominated by national policy and centrally produced documents and analysis, and that they do not necessarily represent what the local level regards as the biggest challenges. In addition, the health profession is a central actor in this planning process and in the partnerships. Thus, HiAP seems to have a relatively high degree of normative legitimacy based on national priorities and scientific knowledge, especially in the health sector, but the extent to which local knowledge is emphasized at the time when health policy is being formulated in municipal plans is variable. The dilemma for HiAP is that people must be mobilized locally, while in practice these strategies are often accomplished based on centrally defined values and perceptions of what is important in public health work (Amdam, 2023).

In the collaboration between MRHT and the municipalities, the dialogs at the strategic level before the pandemic were especially about the long waiting lists for the hospital's and the municipalities' services, and about the unmet needs in society. This is a normative debate about whose needs should be prioritized at any given time and is an ongoing debate where it may prove difficult to point out that some needs are more important than others, especially when it comes to health services. The solution is often to prioritize some needs higher, without other needs being prioritized lower. In any case, such normative debates concern what is important to us, and then conflicts can arise between both governing levels and sectors, and between laymen and scholars.

In a normal situation, the trusts and the municipalities are formally occupied with many tasks, but during the pandemic the most important task was to reduce the spread of infection and to ensure capacity to treat the infected in the health services (Official Norwegian Report, 2021: 6). The health services during COVID-19 were subject to a real danger of overload and resource scarcity. From a situation where almost all needs were prioritized, the purpose now became to prevent the infection from spreading and to treat those who became seriously ill from the infection at the limited intensive hospital places that were available. Other patients had to wait. A national survey carried out by Smedbråten and Thorsager (2020), shows that these patients experienced having received less services during the pandemic both through cancelling appointments and having long-term postponements of planned help and treatment. The survey also points out that several of the respondents reported poorer health and quality of life and that those who have experienced changes in services have largely not been able to participate in the process.

In the autumn of 2020, The Norwegian Directorate of Health established ranked targets for prioritizing vaccines, where reduced risk of death and serious illness was at the top, followed by targets to maintain essential services and critical infrastructure, protect employment and the economy and finally reopen society. A little later, it was prioritized that the elderly and people with underlying diseases should be given priority over the younger ones (Official Norwegian Report, 2023: 16). These prioritizations were quickly perceived as an acceptable norm, but at national level, debates subsequently arose about what provided the most benefit to society and to prioritize the allocation of vaccines to the parts of the country with the highest infection pressure. Here, a social norm and equal distribution were set against local and regional benefits, and in practice the solution became an adaptation of established norm (Christensen & Lægreid, 2023b). In the collaboration in Møre and Romsdal, this debate was not central. Here, the collaboration accepted the strategic prioritization and emphasized agreeing on solutions that were adapted to the local situation.

The virus was new and there was a lack of professional knowledge both at global, national and local level about how the pandemic would develop and how it should be handled. Gradually more knowledge about the virus came, but at the same time new variants and new outbreaks appeared. Christensen and Lægreid (2022b) have found that the crisis management general was not characterized by a scientization of policymaking but became a collaborative decision-making process. Rather than policymaking by experts it became policymaking informed by experts.

As we interpreted our findings, the health professional knowledge was often decisive when the strategic choices were made by the responsible cooperation and crisis management bodies. From the collaboration before the pandemic, some no healthcare personnel had experienced that an emphasis on medical discourse could be exclusionary in the collaboration meeting, but during the pandemic the emphasis on diversity of knowledge and dialogue worked in the collaboration meeting for inclusion and a common understanding of the problem and the solutions. Overall, during the pandemic there was a reasonably good balance between specialist knowledge and local knowledge, and they complemented each other so that the crisis management had high normative legitimacy in relation to a unified understanding of the purpose, and the power to make their own local strategic choices. Not unexpectedly, healthcare knowledge became central. We interpret this to mean that the professionals' recommendations made sense even to those who did not have the professionals' knowledge. This broad opinion-forming process probably affected the first period of the pandemic the most. This suggests that local knowledge was important to legitimize the strategic choices in the early phase of the pandemic, when uncertainty about the pandemic was at its greatest.

The findings indicate that the pandemic meant that HiAP, which until then was largely on the agenda in the municipalities, was put on the agenda both nationally, regionally and locally. There was a common understanding that the pandemic had to be fought. In this sense, the pandemic meant that regional and local pandemic management gained both high normative legitimacy and the power to set the agenda both regionally and locally.

Knowing why. Institutional planning – regulatory legitimacy and power to design the process

Through their respective laws, MRHT and municipalities are required to carry out public health work, and consequently, it must be said that HiAP in Norway today has a high degree of regulative legitimacy (Amdam, 2023). However, this legitimacy reveals an understanding of public health that is in line with what we have here referred to as the conventional and instrumental approach that target individuals and emphasize disease prevention through intervention in lifestyles and influencing the health determinants, which stand in contrast with HiAP as a communicative policymaking process where there are dilemmas and power conflicts. Public health work is a task that belonged to the health sector, and little systematic cooperation with other sectors had been established (Office of the Auditor General, 2015).

The Corona Commission has concluded in its three evaluation reports (Official Norwegian Report, 2021: 6, 2022: 5, 2023: 16) that Norway was not prepared for a pandemic, and that neither were crisis plans prepared or crisis exercises carried out nationally or locally to face a pandemic of the scale that COVID-19 was. Nationally, the people lacked masks, and the healthcare system lacked the necessary infection control equipment for its employees and inadequate crisis plans that had considered such a serious pandemic. When Norwegian society nevertheless turned out to be well equipped to face the pandemic, it is explained by, among other things, a high degree of trust between the people, between the people and the governing authorities, a high level of competence among the people and a good digital infrastructure (Braut, 2023: 65).

Our investigation shows that, in contrast to the national level, the authorities in the county had relevant crisis plans, also for pandemics. Based on experience from serious incidents in the past, for example the Viking Sky accident at Hustavika, the county had both seen the usefulness of good emergency plans, and that the central actors practiced crisis management. Therefore, the institutional design for crisis cooperation at county level during the pandemic was based on plans and exercises. But the established cooperation agreements between MRHT and the municipalities with their formal management structure appear to have gained less importance during COVID-19. MRHT and the municipalities were subject to the national governance, which was more command-oriented during COVID-19 than before the pandemic (Christensen & Lægreid, 2020). The national guidelines for handling the pandemic, seem to have facilitated action where MRHT and the municipalities individually and jointly found solutions to reduce the spread of infection and ensure the capacity of the health services. Overall, the collaboration was adapted to the need for flexibility.

The collaboration processes in the county during COVID-19 can be characterized by common understanding, constant results focus and ability to change. Our informants express that the pandemic work had strong local acceptance, and that there have been some tensions between the national and local governance. An example of this is that the county experienced that there were subsequently many regulatory changes which led to frustrations both in the microbiology services as well as in the company's crisis management. Frustrations were ventilated in the joint meetings in the county, and it was often agreed that "this is how we do it here". This means staying within the laws and regulations but finding local solutions to the challenges.

The management of the crisis in the municipalities, and especially the chief municipal doctors, was not alone. They established contact with colleagues in other municipalities as in the county, with national health authority and institutions, and they were drawn into the collaborative meetings (the Monday meetings and the Tuesday/Wednesday meetings). In this way, the municipalities also achieved a high degree of regulatory legitimacy and power to design the process to handle the pandemic.

The discussions at institutional level before the pandemic between MRHT and the municipalities were mainly process oriented and about the formal collaboration agreement and how they should collaborate. The purpose of HiAP was by no means realized, it only happened when the pandemic ravaged the country. Then the collaboration took on the character of a complete political will formation process. What happened was that the pandemic and the national authorities' handling of it, set new frameworks for the political process. The broad purpose of the health sector was limited to preventing infection and treating the infected, and clear expectations were signalled about what the collaboration should achieve. Collaborative network organizations were established both nationally, regionally and locally which partly built on and partly replaced the existing cooperation.

For the governing bodies and the population, the pandemic became an event that challenged their continued existence. If the governing bodies failed handling the pandemic, questions would subsequently be asked about their existence. If the leaders failed, they could lose their jobs, and if the population did not participate, many could die. The pandemic was quickly perceived as an existential crisis that supported crisis management both nationally, regionally and locally with high regulatory legitimacy and power to set frameworks for and to design the crisis management process itself.

Summary, conclusion and implications

We started this book clarifying the term HiAP and claimed that HiAP is a multi-actor collaboration about policymaking using planning and partnerships as tools. Thus, HiAP represents what we call governance, which is dependent on the formal government's willingness to participate and support. In Chapter 2, we discussed different governing system and their ability to make HiAP successful and we argued that the radical New Public Governance is best suited. This governing system is a reaction against the fragmentation, silo-thinking and unit-egoism that characterize the other governing systems and has the purpose to legitimize political changes and establish more collaboration between involved institutions and actors. In Chapter 3, we discussed how Habermas' political will formation process can be adapted to radical New Public Governance and collaborative planning and become a process supporting HiAP with the needed institutional capacity and democratic legitimacy to succeed. In Chapter 4, we substantiated the will formation process in the ISTOL planning model with relations between the development variables context, mobilization, organizing and implementation, and planning tools institutional, strategic, tactical and operative planning, and in Chapter 5, we discussed how this model can be utilized in monitoring and managing the HiAP as a planning process using the different planning tools to maintain and increase the different forms of democratic legitimacy and institutional capacity. These relations are illustrated with the planning staircase. In this chapter we have used the planning staircase to discuss the democratic legitimacy and institutional capacity of HiAP in three cases. The cases are promoting public health in the BSR (HEPRO), HiAP in Norway before the COVID-19 pandemic, and HiAP in Møre and Romsdal County before and during the pandemic.

The monitoring of HEPRO told us that the condition for collaborative governance was different in the partner countries due to asymmetric power, knowledge and resources, lack of face-to-face dialog and trust between local, regional and national government and lack of facilitating process management, etc. The two other cases told us there as similar lack of conditions in regional and local communities. According to Ansell and Gash (2007) these and other conditions are critical for establishing collaborative governance processes, see Chapter 5. But even if many of the conditions are present, HiAP struggles with establishing a planning process as a complete political will formation process.

In Norway the regulative legitimacy of HiAP is strong, but this does not imply that the normative, cognitive and pragmatic legitimacy in regional and local communities are equally strong. In general, the regional and local planning processes seem to neglect that HiAP is a policymaking process that must continuously try to increase HiAP's democratic legitimacy and institutional capacity. And as a governance structure HiAP need to become a counterforce that demands changes in the fragmented government structure. It is commonly recognized that governance lives in the shadow of governance and that realizing HiAP as a multi-actor approach need participation and support from the different government sectors and levels.

Before the COVID-19 pandemic the government actors had almost not been held accountable for the lack of outcome and impacts regarding improving public health. This changed dramatically during the pandemic because the pandemic become an existential crisis with potential negative effects both on the people in charge and on the population if the handling of the crisis failed. Even if Norway was not properly prepared for a pandemic, collaborative planning and partnerships were early established at national, regional and local level during the crisis. A clear mission was formulated at national level, and the whole government and the inhabitants were kept accountable for fulfilling it. The pandemic led to the establishment of a complete communicative planning process that gave crisis management high democratic legitimacy and institutional capacity for action. Handling the crisis became Health in All Policies with the characteristic of policy formulation in arenas with broad participation, dialogue and a large degree of equality, and a process where planning and partnership became important tools. The pandemic forced the HiAP practice to become radical New Public Management which delivered activities with efficiency, effectiveness, quality and legitimacy and which sustained HiAP with high democratic legitimacy and institutional power.

In this new practice the local and regional leaders participated with their competences and through the sharing of knowledge that took place in the collaboration in the county and the municipalities. Those involved developed common knowledge about why the handling of the pandemic was necessary, what was most important to grasp, how to proceed and to translate the common knowledge into actions. Through face-to-face dialogue, the actors' values, knowledge, skills and abilities were exposed in the critical reflections. Many actors stood out as competent leaders, and the collaborative bodies functioned as competence building processes for those involved. In this process inhabitants became active citizens and took responsibility for their own and other's health. The inhabitants became co-creators when they restricted their travelling, respected distance to other people, cleaned their hands, etc.

These conclusions support our argumentation in this book that HiAP depends on the practice of radical New Public Governance to succeed. Now after the pandemic, the big question is what the actors locally and regionally will bring into the wider collaboration, and what new structures and processes will be established to promote collaboration to improve people's health. Many informants say they have learned a lot during the process, but we would say that it is an open question what they take with them to the normal situation, since the pandemic had such a clear impression of being an exceptional situation.

So, what implication can be drawn. First of all HiAP need to be practice as radical New Public Governance with a complete political will formation process with collaborative planning and partnerships. This implies handling HiAP as we handled COVID-19. The first step towards realizing this must be to supplement the national legislations which give the HiAP input legitimacy, with an accountability system demanding the government to get out of their silos and engage in collaborative planning and partnerships with their competence. Accountability design has so far not been a central part of collaborative governance arrangements. The purpose must be to increase the outcome legitimacy by delivering health actions with high regulative legitimacy regarding overall societal values as democracy, equality, sustainability and public health, in addition to high normative, cognitive and pragmatic legitimacy. A second step must be to change the role of the inhabitants from mainly clients, users and co-producers of health services, to active co-creators of their health. However, HiAP need to be legitimized top-down and bottom-up simultaneous in a political will forming process, and collaborative planning and partnerships can be the tool. In this way the problematic duality between legitimacy and action can be solved, and increased democratic legitimacy can support HiAP with institutional capacity to act.

References

Amdam, R. 2010. *Planning in Health Promotion Work: an Empowerment Model.* Abingdon, Oxon and New York: Routledge.

Amdam, R. 2011. *Planlegging og prosessleiing. Korleis lykkast i utviklingsarbeid.* Oslo: Samlaget.

Amdam, R. 2023. "Health in All Policies" in Norwegian municipalities—Dilemmas and lack of legitimacy and capacity. *International Journal of Health Planning and Management*, 38: 1345–1359. http://dx.doi.org/10.1002/hpm.3664

Amdam, R., Larsen, A. S. A., Nerland, S. M. K. & Teige, B. K. 2025 (work in progress). *Koronapandemien sine mange ansikt: historier frå lokale krisesamarbeid.* Oslo: Universitetsforlaget.

Ansell, C. & Gash, A. 2007. Collaborative governance in theory and practice. *Journal of Public Administration Research and Theory*, 18 (4): 543–571. https://doi:10.1093/jopart/mum032

Braut, G. S. 2023. Kva lærte me eigentleg av pandemien? *Michael.* 2023, 20 (1), 64–74. https://hvlopen.brage.unit.no/hvlopen-xmlui/handle/11250/3069719

Capano, G., Howlett, M., Jarvis, D. S. L., Ramesh, M. & Goyal, N. 2020. Mobilizing policy capacity to fight COVID-19: Understanding variations in state responses. *Policy and Society*, 39 (3): 285–308. https://doi.org/10.1080/14494035.2020.1787628

Christensen, T. & Lægreid, P. 2004. *The Fragmented State – the Challenges of Combining Efficiency, Institutional Norms and Democracy.* Working paper 3 – 2004. Bergen: Stein Rokkan Centre for Social Studies. https://norceresearch.brage.unit.no/norceresearch-xmlui/bitstream/handle/1956/1369/N03-04%5B1%5D.pdf

Christensen, T. & Lægreid, P. 2020. Balancing governance capacity and legitimacy: How the Norwegian Government handled the COVID-19 crisis as a high performer. *Public Administration Review*, 80 (5): 774–779. https://doi.org/10.1111/puar.13241

Christensen, T. & Lægreid, P. 2022a. Norway: A pragmatic, collaborative, and legitimate response. In: Lynggaard, K., Jensen, M. D. & Kluth, M. (eds.) *Governments' Responses to the Covid-19 Pandemic in Europe*: 295–306. Cham: Palgrave Macmillan. https://doi.org/10.1007/978-3-031-14145-4_25

Christensen, T. & Lægreid, P. 2022b. Scientization under pressure—The problematic role of expert bodies during the handling of the COVID-19 pandemic. *Public Organization Review* (22): 291–307. https://doi.org/10.1007/s11115-022-00605-0

Christensen, T. & Lægreid, P. 2023a. Crisis management of the COVID-19: The Nordic Way and Swedish exceptionalism. In: Cheung, A. B. L. & Thiel, S. V. (eds.) *Crisis Leadership and Public Governance during the COVID–19 Pandemic*: 289–323. Singapore: World Scientific Publishing. http://dx.doi.org/10.1142/9789811262852_0011

Christensen, T. & Lægreid, P. 2023b. The politics of vaccines—How to determine a fair vaccine allocation: Hierarchy, negotiations, or culture? *Administration & Society*, 55 (6): 1–23. https://doi.org/10.1177/00953997231167557

Friedmann, J. 1992. *Empowerment. The Politics of Alternative Development.* Cambridge MA and Oxford UK: Blackwell Publishers.

Friedmann, J. & Weaver, C. 1979. *Territory and Function. The Evolution of Regional Planning*. London: Edward Arnold.

Giddens, A. 1984. *The Constitutions of Society: Outline of the Theory of Structuration.* Berkeley CA: University of California Press.

Giddens, A. 1990. *The Consequences of Modernity*. Stanford CA: Stanford University Press.

Habermas, J. 1996. *Between Facts and Norms: Contributions to a Discourse Theory of Law and Democracy*. Massachusetts and London: MIT Press.

Jessop, B. 1997. A neo-Gramscian approach to the regulation of urban regimes: Accumulation strategies, hegemonic projects, and governance. In: Lauria, M. (ed.) *Reconstructing Urban Regime Theory: Regulating Urban Politics in a Global Economy*: 51–73. London: Sage.

Lægreid, P. & Rykkja, L. H. 2022. Accountability and inter- organizational collaboration within the state. *Public Management Review*, 24:5, 683–703. https://doi.org/10.1080/14719037.2021.1963822
Lund-Tønnesen, J. & Christensen, T. 2023. Learning from the COVID-19 pandemic: Implications from governance capacity and legitimacy. *Public Organization Review*. https://doi.org/10.1007/s11115-023-00705-5
Ministry of Health and Care, 2019. Avtale mellom regjeringen og KS om innføring av helsefellesskap for å skape en mer sammenhengende helse- og omsorgstjeneste. https://www.regjeringen.no/contentassets/77ad51af47bf4711923fa82a0899daff/191023_helsefellesskap_avtale.pdf
Nicola, R. M. & Hatcher, M. T. 2000. A framework for building effective public health constituencies. *Public Health Management Practice*, 6 (2): 1–10. https://doi.org/10.1097/00124784-200006020-00003
Nylenna, M. 2014. *Helsetjenesten i Norge. Et overblikk*. Gyldendal akademisk.
Office of the Auditor General 2015. The office of the auditor General's investigation of public health work. *Document*, 3: 11. (2014–2015). Oslo.
Official Norwegian Report. 2021: 6. *The authorities' handling of the coronavirus pandemic*. https://www.regjeringen.no/no/dokumenter/horing-nou-2021-6-myndighetenes-handtering-av-koronapandemien/id2846977/
Official Norwegian Report. 2022: 5. *The authorities' handling of the coronavirus pandemic*. Part 2. https://www.regjeringen.no/no/dokumenter/nou-2022-5/id2910055/
Official Norwegian Report. 2023: 16. *The authorities' handling of the coronavirus pandemic*. https://www.regjeringen.no/no/dokumenter/horing-nou-2023-16-evaluering-av-pandemihandteringen-rapport-fra-koronautvalget/id2985289/
Østfold County Council 2005. *The HEPRO-project plan*. Sarpsborg: Østfold County Council.
Rohde, T., Grut, L., Lippestad, J. & Anthun, K. 2020. *Samhandling mellom og kommuner – før og etter samhandlingsreformen. Tidsskrift for Omsorgsforskning*, 6(3), 1–17. https://doi.org/10.18261/issn.2387-5984-2020-03-05
Rommetvedt, H. 2021. Samarbeidsutvalgene mellom kommuner og helseforetak: Arena for maktkamp eller forum for deliberasjon? *Norsk statsvitenskapelig tidsskrift*, 37(2), 116–132. https://doi.org/10.18261/issn.1504-2936-2021-02-03
Rommetvedt, H. & Nødland, S. I. 2020. *Samarbeidsavtalene mellom helseforetak kommuner og sykehus*. Oslo: SINTEF Digital Rapport. https://www.ks.no/contentassets/37b511d26ff94bc9bb200538ecba4430/Samhandling-mellom-kommuner-og-sykehus.pdf
Smedbråten, K. & Thorsager, M. 2020. *Pasient-og brukererfaringer med tjenester under koronapandemien 2020*. S. Helsetilsyn. https://www.helsetilsynet.no/globalassets/opplastinger/publikasjoner/rapporter2020/helsetilsynetrapport6_2020.pdf
Ståhl, T., Wismar, M., Ollila, E., Lahtinen, E., Melkas, T. & Leppo, K. 2006. *Health in All Policies: Prospects and Potentials*. Ministry of Social Affairs and Health. https://ec.europa.eu/health/ph_projects/2005/action1/docs/2005_1_18_frep_a4_en.pdf
Stöhr, W. 1990. Synthesis, introduction and on the theory and practice of local development in Europe. In: Stöhr, W. (ed.) *Global Challenge and Local Response*. London and New York: Mansell.
Svendsen, G. T. & Svendsen, G. L. H. 2006. *Social kapital. En introduktion*. København: Hans Reitzels.

INDEX